TREATISE ON REVIEW ARTICLES IN NURSING

DR. V. HEMAVATHY

RIGI PUBLICATION

Treatise on Review Articles in Nursing

BY

Dr. V. Hemavathy

Originally published in India

ISBN: 978-93-95773-17-1

Published by RIGI PUBLICATION

777, Street no.9, Krishna Nagar

Khanna-141401 (Punjab), India

Website: www.rigipublication.com

Email: info@rigipublication.com

Phone: +91-9357710014, +91-9465468291

CONTENTS

Nat. Volatiles & Essent. Oils, 2021; 8(4): 1-9

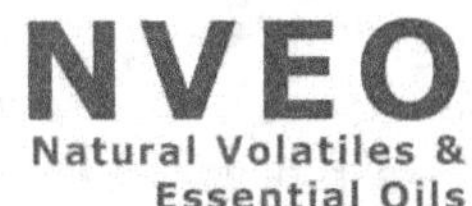

An illness that attack your brain and nerve cells -Parkinson's plus syndromes

[1] Dr.V.HEMAVATHY, [2] DR. JOHNSON WMS

[1]*Principal, Sree Balaji College of Nursing, Bharath Institute of Higher Education and Research, Chennai, Tamil Nadu, India*

[2]*Dean, Sree Balaji Medical College and Hospital, Bharath Institute of Higher Education and Research, Chennai, Tamil Nadu, India*

Abstract

Parkinson's plus syndromesare illnesses that attack your brain and nerve cells. As the name suggests, they're linked to Parkinson's disease and cause a lot of the same symptoms, but they can bring on other problems as well. Brain makes a chemical called dopamine that helps control your movement. Parkinson's disease is by far the most common of these, but about 15% of people who have a problem making dopamine will have one of the Parkinson's plus syndromes.Parkinson's plus syndromes are more serious and harder to treat than "classic" Parkinson's disease. The four main types are:Progressive Supranuclear Palsy (PSP),Dementia with Lewy Bodies,Multiple System Atrophy and Corticobasal Degeneration

Keywords: Parkinson plus syndrome, dopamine, movement

Introduction

Parkinson's plus syndromes, also called "atypical Parkinson's," are illnesses that attack your brain and nerve cells. As the name suggests, they're linked to Parkinson's disease and cause a lot of the same symptoms, but they can bring on other problems as well. Brain makes a chemical called dopamine that helps control your movement. Parkinson's disease is by far the most common of these, but about 15% of people who have a problem making dopamine will have one of the Parkinson's plus syndromes.

Researchers aren't sure what causes Parkinson's or Parkinson's plus syndrome. There might be some genetic or environmental risk factors that can increase the likelihood of developing Parkinson's plus syndrome. For example, some scientists theorize that exposure to toxins could cause your risk, but more research needs to be done to prove this link.

Types

Parkinson's plus syndromes are more serious and harder to treat than "classic" Parkinson's disease. The four main types are:

Progressive Supranuclear Palsy (PSP)

This is the most common Parkinson's plus syndrome. It causes some of the same issues with movement and your muscles as Parkinson's disease, like stiffness and problems with walking or balance, but it doesn't usually make your limbs shake. It also can make it harder to move your eyes -- it starts in the part of your brain that controls your eye muscles. Looking down can be especially hard. It can cause mood changes, affect your ability to think of words, and make it hard to swallow as well. PSP causes trouble with balance and stability that can mimic Parkinson's disease. Unlike Parkinson's disease, people with PSP don't experience tremors. They do have difficulty with eye movement and are likely to experience more trouble with speech, swallowing, and mood than people with Parkinson's disease.

Dementia With Lewy Bodies

LBD is a progressive brain condition caused by structures called Lewy bodies that form in your brain. People with LBD might have symptoms that resemble Parkinson's disease, dementia, or a combination of both. This is the second most common form of dementia after Alzheimer's disease. Lewy bodies are clumps of protein that build up in your nerve cells. When that happens, it affects your ability to think clearly, speak, and remember things. It can make you confused and cause hallucinations (when you see things that aren't there). The symptoms get worse over time.

Multiple System Atrophy

MSA is a progressive condition that affects your nervous system. It causes stiffness and loss of balance similarly to Parkinson's disease. Over time, the effects of the disease on your nervous system can lead to difficulty with essential body functions such as digestion, breathing, and your heartbeat. This affects what's known as your autonomic nervous system, which controls things like your blood pressure and digestive system. Symptoms can include things like fainting, losing control of your bladder, and constipation. It also causes more typical Parkinson's symptoms, like shaking, stiffness, and problems with balance or speech. MSA is a progressive condition that affects your nervous system. It causes stiffness and loss of balance similarly to Parkinson's disease. Over time, the effects of the disease on your nervous system can lead to difficulty with essential body functions such as digestion, breathing, and your heartbeat.

Corticobasal Degeneration

It is a condition that causes parts of your brain to become smaller. This causes many symptoms that overlap with Parkinson's disease, such as tremors and balance problems. Over time, it can lead to difficulty with both speaking and writing.

This is the rarest of the four main types. It kills brain cells in the cerebral cortex -- the wrinkly grey matter on the outside of your brain -- and causes the cortex to shrink. It also attacks what's called the basal ganglia, a part of your brain that controls movement.

Its symptoms are like the ones caused by Parkinson's disease, including the loss of muscle control, sometimes starting on only one side of your body. But it also can hurt your ability to think, see, and speak clearly. As the disease gets worse, it gets harder to walk and swallow. CBGD is a condition that causes parts of your brain to become smaller. This causes many symptoms that overlap with

Parkinson's disease, such as tremors and balance problems. Over time, it can lead to difficulty with both speaking and writing.

Unique symptoms of PSP include:

- falling backward
- blurred vision and difficulty reading
- difficulty moving the eyes up and down
- slurred speech
- difficulty swallowing
- depression or other mood issues
- behavioural changes
- laughing or crying at inappropriate times

Unique symptoms of MSA include:

- breathing problems that get worse at night
- syncope, or passing out
- dizziness
- slurred speech
- low blood pressure
- bladder problems
- sleep disturbances

Unique symptoms of CBGD include:

- one-sided movement trouble
- involuntary muscle contractions
- rapid muscle jerks
- trouble with concentration
- trouble with communication
- behavioural changes

- trouble coordinating movements, or apraxia
- loss of control over an arm called "alien limb syndrome"

Unique symptoms of LBD include:

- difficulty processing information
- difficulty following instructions
- decreased awareness of surroundings
- hallucinations
- delusions
- sleep disturbances
- mood changes

Other things that can point to a Parkinson's plus syndrome rather than the classic form include:

- Early signs of dementia
- Falling often
- Trouble moving your eyes
- Your symptoms get worse then level off for a while

Diagnosis

Parkinson's plus syndromes can look a lot like other conditions that affect your nervous system, so it can sometimes take a while to find out for sure what's going on.

If your doctor thinks you might have Parkinson's or a Parkinson's plus syndrome, they'll recommend that you see a neurologist, a doctor who specializes in problems with the nervous system. Your neurologist will examine you and see how you move and follow directions. They then might suggest blood tests and a brain scan to rule out other conditions.

If those don't show a reason for your symptoms, they may ask you to try a medication called carbidopa-levodopa. Your brain can turn that into dopamine. If your symptoms get better, that may be enough for your doctor to diagnose Parkinson's disease. If it doesn't help much or at all, or it helps for a while then stops working that can be a sign of a Parkinson's plus syndrome.

Treatment

Doctors don't know exactly what causes any of the Parkinson's plus syndromes, and there's no cure for them. Treating them usually is about managing the symptoms. That can include the following:

- Medication can help some people move more easily and feel less stiff. Some drugs also can help with the problems caused by multiple system atrophy, like fainting or constipation.
- A cane or walker can help you get around.
- Speech therapy can help you communicate better.
- Exercise and physical therapy can make your muscles stronger and more flexible.
- Occupational therapy can help make everyday tasks easier.

Parkinson's plus syndrome is the name for a group of neurological conditions that are very similar to Parkinson's disease. Because these conditions cause symptoms that are very similar to Parkinson's, they are often incorrectly diagnosed. However, these conditions can even be treated using many of the same medications and therapies as Parkinson's.

The symptoms of Parkinson have plus can vary and depend on the condition you have. Many people will have symptoms that are also found in Parkinson's disease, such as:

- balance problems
- tremors
- stiffness or muscle rigidity
- difficulty walking and standing
- difficulty controlling your movements
- fatigue
- confusion

The conditions that make up Parkinson's plus are not actually Parkinson's disease and do have unique symptoms.

People with Parkinson's plus syndrome are often diagnosed with Parkinson's disease in the early years of their condition. However, their condition won't progress like Parkinson's disease. It might progress faster, and they might start to develop symptoms that aren't present in Parkinson's disease.

There is no definitive test for Parkinson's or Parkinson's plus syndrome. Instead, a doctor might conduct a series of tests that will look at your balance, ability to walk, and coordination. These are generally simple in-office tests involving the doctor watching you walk, sit, stand, and perform other movements. You'll likely also do some memory and cognition tests with the doctor.

The doctor might also order some imaging tests to get a closer look at your brain. These may include:

- **MRI scan.** An MRI uses magnetic waves to create images of your body.
- **PET scan.** A PET scan uses a special dye to look for damage to your brain.
- **CT.** A CT scan can check your brain activity.

What causes it?

Researchers aren't sure what causes Parkinson's or Parkinson's plus syndrome. There might be some genetic or environmental risk factors that can increase the likelihood of developing Parkinson's plus syndrome. For example, some scientists theorize that exposure to toxins could cause your risk, but more research needs to be done to prove this link.

Although the underlying cause isn't known, we do know what changes to your body can cause each Parkinson's plus syndrome:

- **PSP.** When you have PSP, a build-up of protein in your brain cells causes them to deteriorate. Your condition will progress as this continues.
- **MSA.** As with PSP, proteins accumulate in the cells of your brain that control your central nervous system and other vital functions.
- **CBGD.** A protein called tau builds up in your brain cells when you have CBGD. This build up causes the symptoms of CBGD.
- **LBD.** Protein clusters called Lewy bodies grow in your brain when you have LBD. Over time, the Lewy bodies cause changes to your brain that impact your ability to function.

What are the current treatment options?

While there is no specific cure for Parkinson's plus syndrome, there are treatments that can control your symptoms. A doctor can develop a plan for your overall health and to treat your specific symptoms. Medications that treat the symptoms of Parkinson's disease often do not work as well for Parkinson's plus syndrome.

Treatment options might include:

- **Walking and balance assistance.** You might receive physical and occupational therapy to help keep you moving. Therapists can help you build strength and prevent falls. They can also help you learn to use canes, walkers, and other mobility aids, if needed.
- **Swallowing and speech assistance.** A speech therapist can help you adjust to changes that might make it hard to swallow and speak. They can help you communicate and can recommend foods and beverages that are easier to swallow.
- **Medications for cognitive issues.** Your doctor might prescribe a variety of medications that can help with your focus and memory. Many of these medications are also used for conditions such

as Alzheimer's or dementia.

- **Medications for trouble with movement.** You might be prescribed medications that can help you control your muscles and movement. These medications might also address stiffness and balance problems.
- **Medications to help with mood symptoms.** If you're experiencing depression, anxiety, or other mood-related concerns, your doctor might prescribe medications that can help with these symptoms.

What's the outlook for people with Parkinson's plus?

Although there currently isn't a treatment to halt the progression of Parkinson's plus syndrome, there are treatments that can help you manage your symptoms and improve your quality of life.

The exact outlook for Parkinson's plus syndrome depends on the person and the specific condition they have. Someone who is otherwise healthy when they're diagnosed will typically have a longer life expectancy than someone who is already facing other health conditions when they're diagnosed. Your doctor will monitor your condition over time and can let you know how it's progressing.

Treatment

No cures currently exist for atypical Parkinsonism. The goal of treatment is to manage symptoms for as long as possible. The appropriate medication for each disorder depends on your symptoms and how you respond to treatment.

For LBD, some people find relief from symptoms with cholinesterase inhibitors. These drugs increase the activity of neurotransmitters that affect memory and judgment.

For PSP, levodopa and similar drugs that act like dopamine, are helpful for some people.

Participating in physical or occupational therapy can also help with most of these conditions. Keeping physically active may help relieve symptoms. Check with your doctor if any specific exercises might be good for you.

Risk factors

Certain risk factors are known for PD, but little has been established for atypical Parkinsonism. The known risk factors for PD include:

- **Advancing age.** This is the most common risk factor for PD.
- **Biological sex.** Those assigned male at birth tend to develop PD more often than those assigned female at birth.
- **Genetics.** Many studies are exploring the genetic link to PD.

- **Environmental causes.** A variety of toxins have been linked to PD.
- **Head trauma.** Injuries to the brain are thought to contribute to PD onset.

Much research is ongoing to establish risk factors for atypical Parkinsonism disorders, especially in genetics.

Some atypical Parkinsonism disorders have obvious risk factors. For example, drug-induced Parkinsonism is related to certain drugs, and vascular Parkinsonism stems from previous strokes.

But the risk factors for the other Parkinsonisms are the subject of a lot of current research. Scientists are looking into why each of these conditions occur and how to slow or stop their progression.

Possible complications

Perhaps the most serious complication from any of these conditions is dementia.

You may first develop mild cognitive impairment (MCI), which may not interfere too much with your daily activities. If your thinking skills and memory gradually decline, you may need the assistance of family, a home health aide, or an assisted living facility.

Because these conditions affect balance and coordination, fall risk becomes an important concern. Having PD or atypical Parkinsonism means avoiding falls and fractures. Make your home safer by getting rid of throw rugs, lighting hallways at night, and installing grab bars in the bathroom.

Atypical Parkinsonian syndromes are progressive diseases. This means that their symptoms will continue to worsen over time. While no cures exist for these disorders yet, there are treatments that can help to slow their progression.

It's important that you take your medications exactly as prescribed by your doctor. If you're ever unsure about your treatment, call your doctor's office.

PD and atypical Parkinsonism affect each person differently. Those differences include the type and severity of symptoms, as well as life expectancy.

One study found that assuming an average age of about 72 years at diagnosis, people with atypical Parkinsonism lived on average 6 more years.

Life expectancy estimates can vary greatly depending on your overall health. The healthier you are when you're diagnosed, the better your chances of living longer with atypical Parkinsonism.

Conclusion

Patients with Parkinsonism-plus syndromes represent a relatively small portion of Parkinsonism patients seen in general and movement disorders clinics. Given the wide spectrum of disease phenotypes associated with these disorders and the often subtle clinical differences, establishing the correct diagnosis, especially at disease onset, can be difficult despite serial clinical observations and repeated neurological examination. Autopsy confirmation is often necessary. Advancement in molecular genetics may provide a better understanding of some of these rare syndromes and holds substantial promise for more rational classification and therapy. Moreover, an accurate diagnosis of these disorders is necessary to understand their cause and pathogenesis. This may allow development of biologic therapeutic strategies to stop or slow disease progression, such as inhibition of tau or a-synuclein aggregation.

REFERENCES

Mitra K, Gangopadhaya PK, Das SK. Parkinsonism plus syndrome: a review. Neurol India. 2003; 51 (2): p.183-188.

Vanacore N, Bonifati V, Fabbrini G, et al. Epidemiology of multiple system atrophy. Neurological Sciences. 2001; 22 (1): p.97-99. doi: 10.1007/s100720170064 . | Open in Read by QxMD

Hot cross bun sign (pons). https://radiopaedia.org/articles/hot-cross-bun-sign-pons. Updated: January 1, 2017. Accessed: July 13, 2017.

Ahmed Z, Asi YT, Sailer A, et al. The neuropathology, pathophysiology and genetics of multiple system atrophy. Neuropathol Appl Neurobiol. 2012; 38 (1): p.4- 24. doi: 10.1111/j.1365-2990.2011.01234.x . | Open in Read by QxMD

Booth TC, Nathan M, Waldman AD, Quigley AM, Schapira AH, Buscombe J. The Role of Functional Dopamine-Transporter SPECT Imaging in Parkinsonian Syndromes, Part 2. Am J Neuroradiol. 2014 . doi: 10.3174/ajnr.A3971 . | Open in Read by QxMD

Pure Autonomic Failure. http://www.merckmanuals.com/professional/neurologic-disorders/autonomic-nervous-system/pure-autonomic-failure. Updated: March 1, 2017. Accessed: July 5, 2017.

Multiple System Atrophy Fact Sheet. https://www.ninds.nih.gov/Disorders/Patient- Caregiver-Education/Fact-Sheets/Multiple-System-Atrophy. Updated: April 22, 2020. Accessed: December 28, 2020.

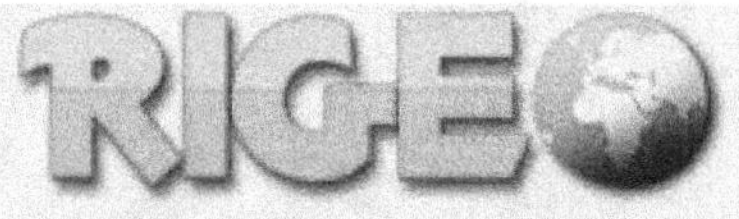

www.rigeo.org **REVIEW OF INTERNATIONAL GEOGRAPHICAL EDUCATION**

ISSN: 2146-0353 • © RIGEO • 11(10), SPRING, 2021

www.rigeo.org Research Article

THE TERRIBLE TOLL OF COVID-19 ON PEOPLE WITH INTELLECTUAL DISABILITIES

DR.V.HEMAVATHY
PRINCIPAL
SREE BALAJI COLLEGE OF NURSING
BHARATH INSTITUTE OF HIGHER EDUCATION
AND RESEARCH

DR.S.BHUMINATHAN
REGISTRAR
BHARATH INSTITUTE OF HIGHER EDUCATION
AND RESEARCH

Abstract

In the wake of the COVID19 epidemic, everyone will be affected. As a result of the epidemic, people with intellectual disabilities (IDs) are more susceptible to its physical, mental, and social effects. When cognitive deficiencies limit their ability to comprehend information, they must rely on guardians to keep an eye on them while they are quarantined. Individuals on the autistic spectrum may become more defiant, which might increase their risk of dislocation and their need on psychiatric medications if their regular activities are curtailed. Individual communities no longer safeguard identified persons, leaving them open to exploitation by others. In the event of future pandemics, the impact of COVID19 on peoplewith IDs should be taken into consideration. People with ID and those who care for them will be betterprepared to deal with future epidemics of infectious diseases if evidence is gathered in a methodicalmanner.

Keywords: Autism, COVID-19, intellectual disability, pandemic

To cite this article: DR.V.HEMAVATHY and DR.S.BHUMINATHAN. (2021) THE TERRIBLE TOLL OF COVID-19 ON PEOPLE WITH INTELLECTUAL DISABILITIES *(RIGEO), 11*(10), XXXX-XXXX. doi: 10.48047/rigeo.11.10.XXXX

Submitted: 09-10-2020 • **Revised:** 11-12-2020 • **Accepted:** 13-02-2021

INTRODUCTION:

COVID-19 is six times more likely to kill patients with intellectual disability than the general population. During the pandemic and in the future, an expert tells us what we need to do to improve their treatment. Millions of individuals have been infected by the global epidemic of COVID19, which has spread fast over the world. In the wake of the pandemic, it became clear that certain categories of people were particularly vulnerable. Mental health issues, substance abuse, and social exclusion plague people with intellectual disabilities (IDs), making them particularly vulnerable. Health care providers face a problem in protecting persons with ID against infection and assisting those who have been afflicted. When a person's particular features allow him or her to adapt to new situations, he or she might create new services. Families and caregivers are concerned that people with disabilities may be overlooked during the epidemic and that the response should not exclude them(Belingheri, Paladino, & Riva, 2020).

In the present pandemic of the Coronavirus, people with ID are at a greater risk than the general population of people. To put it another way, people with ID have underlying health concerns that make them more vulnerable to the pandemic, which means they're more likely to wind up at nursing homes and other communal settings that have been at the centre of the spread of the disease. Both family carers and those who work for providers are under a great deal of strain because of their caregiving duties. Many Direct Support Professionals (DSPs) who work with persons with disabilities provide services that can't be done from a distance of six feet. DSPs confront many of the same difficulties and dangers as health care workers, but often lack the PPE and supplies necessary to provide safe care to people with I/DD who are confined or shelteringin their homes.

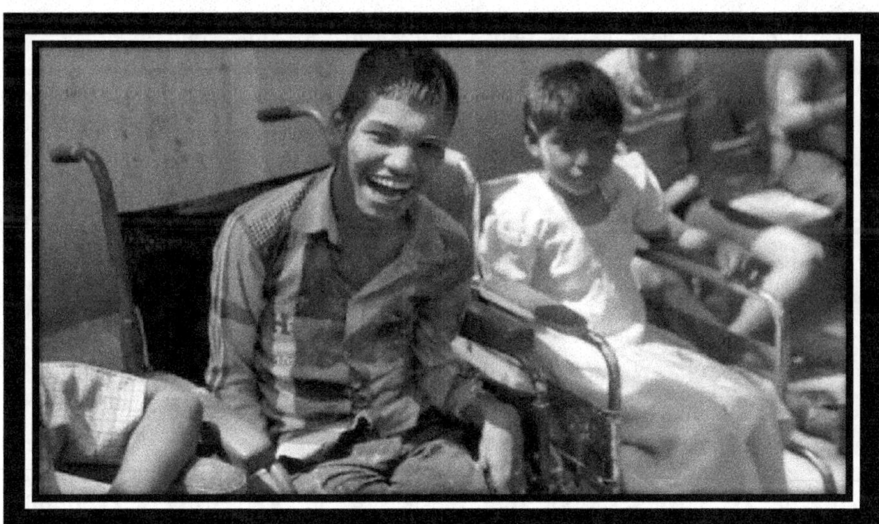

TODAY'S MAJOR CHALLENGES, AS WELL AS THOSE WE HAVE IDENTIFIED, :

A shortage of Personal Protective Equipment (PPE) is affecting the DSP workforce and service providers' ability to keep employees and people with disabilities safe. DSPs, like healthcare professionals, undertake vital job but lack the supplies they require. A decrease in the number of services that help people with disabilities integrate into their communities is a major problem for them. In a world they may not comprehend or be able to cope with, people with disabilities are being further isolated. They need physical, emotional, and behavioural help. There are many students with disabilities who are unable to participate in remote schooling due to a lack of support. Violence and abuse are more likely to occur when people feel isolated and stressed.

DAY SUPPORTS – More than 620,000 persons with ID are receiving day programmes andemployment services, and thousands more are eligible but are not currently receiving them. All day programmes have been shut down in most states, and more states are expected to followsuit. People with ID are being kept apart from the rest of the population in their homes. For some,this involves a group home, while for others, it's their own home.

RESIDENTIAL SUPPORTS– Over 680,000 persons with ID live in some sort of supported housing, more than 790,000 live alone or with a roommate, and thousands more are eligible for assistancebut are on waiting lists for them. They are currently sheltering in place for persons with ID who live in group homes or other assisted residences, and for those who are on their own. It's a full-time job for local chapters of The Arc and other providers to give 24-hour support for these residents, including assisting in their knowledge of the epidemic and providing for their daily needs, like as personal care and meals.

FAMILY SUPPORTS– More than 3.6 million people in the United States have an I.D. that allows them to remain at their primary residence. Family caregivers are being forced to quit their employment in order to stay at home with their loved ones with ID who can't be left alone as a result of the shutdown of numerous day care centres and schools. Many family members are unable to leave the house to buy groceries, pick up medications, or obtain other necessities because they lack the resources to do so. They face many of the same challenges and hazards as group home caregivers in terms of safety, emotional and behavioural assistance, and addressing fundamental human needs. Unemployment and job losses are also hurting familycaregivers' ability to support their loved ones with ID.

HOSPITAL TREATMENT – Families and loved ones of people with I/DD worry about how they will be treated in the hospital. They are worried that in the event of a scarcity of ventilators, medication, or other life-saving care, they may be denied access due to discriminatory restrictions in state health department and hospital planning documents. They are concerned about the lack of support they require to interact successfully with their doctors. Family members, DSPs, and otherdisability service providers may not be allowed in the patient's room to help communicate with medical experts making key treatment decisions because of the necessity to confine the virus andthe shortage of PPE.

RISK OF INFECTION

For a variety of reasons, such as physical health issues, societal roots, and cognitive impairments,those who have been identified are at greater risk of infection. ID patients had greater rates ofconcomitant somatic disorders and a lower life expectancy than the general population, with a mortality rate of 3.18 per 100,000. People having genetic abnormalities that can be passed downfrom generation to generation, such as metabolic congenital heart defects or respiratory ailmentsIn persons with ID, respiratory tract infections are the primary cause of death. People with ID are more likely to be obese, which raises the risk of COVID19 infections.

The amount of money granted to people with ID who live in the community with the help of afamily member or carer is usually based on how much assistance they require. People with mild cognitive impairment (IQ 50-70) may require less support than those with moderate to severe cognitive impairment. They have easy access to community activities because of their involvement in them, and some even get compensated for their efforts. The habits of people withIDs can vary, therefore they must be prepared for that. Changes like this can make you moreanxious, which can lead to behavioural issues and underlying mental illnesses..

RESPONDING TO THE PANDEMIC FOR PEOPLE WITH ID

Shortly after the call for help from individuals and caregivers, non-governmental organisations (NGOs) prepared materials on COVID19 and for those with ID. For persons with IDs who are unable to speak for themselves, volunteer organisations have been successful in raising public awarenessof their condition and addressing preconceptions. It was originally proposed that the ClinicalHazard Scale be used to determine a patient's appropriateness for more intrusive therapies byNICE guidelines, NG159. Denying them medical care due to their incapacity will help you savemoney.

SUPPORT FOR THOSE INFECTED WITH COVID19

In many nations, the extent of transmission of the virus is unknown because of a lack of strategic and proactive testing for the virus in general. living in groups of people Only a few studies have been done on the prevalence of infection among patients with ID in the community and in hospitals. Care for an infected person requires the use of personal protective equipment (PPE) and knowledge of infection control procedures. If caregivers want to help patients stay in thecommunity, they must learn new skills that nurses frequently practise and perform. As a precautionary measure, measures such as fencing and infection control should be used. Whenemployees are unable to work because of illness or the urge for self-isolation, services can suffer.There is a global scarcity of personal protective equipment (PPE) for caregivers, as suggested by (Belingheri et al., 2020).

ADVANCE HEALTH PLANNING

Caregivers and family members face a difficult tzask while preparing to care for those at high risk of mortality. Families and people with intellectual disabilities (ID) can better prepare for this eventuality with the support of early care planning. Caregivers can also ask children and teensabout their thoughts and wants regarding hospice care.

THE IMPACT ON FAMILIES AND CARERS

Family and caregivers are particularly affected by the pandemic when the typical supports ofresidential schools, day services, or respite care are no longer available. Local authorities andgovernment entities are needed to help families cope with the hardship of providing 24-hour carethat was formerly provided by paid caregivers. As a result of this, families' finances and well-beingand mental health would be affected. Families are at risk of a collapse if they don't receive more care, which could lead to a hospitalisation because of their children's increasingly troublesomebehaviour (Moghadas et al., 2020).
Some people's mental health may be affected by social isolation and quarantine measures in place, in addition to the stress caused by the dread of getting the sickness(Burcelin, Courtney, & Amar, 2015).Individuals with ID may be affected in the same way, if not more so, because of the demands of quarantine that may lead to maladaptive behaviours. Autism or ADHD in someonewith ID may make the condition even worse if their daily routines are disrupted and their physical surroundings is limited (Jm, 2010). The disintegration of a person's care network and the consequent worsening of behavioural problems can occur if carers of people with ID isolate themselves.

Exceptional events like the current lockdown can lead to an increase in anxiety and paranoia. When it comes to COVID-19, people with ID and autism may become preoccupied, which is unsurprising considering the prevalence of obsessional thinking and obsessive compulsive behaviours in the autistic spectrum population(Crawley et al., 2020).Anxiety and paranoia may result in behavioural issues as a result of this. Comorbid OCD may be worsened by an obsessive-compulsive desire for personal hygiene. These stressors can lead to mental disease if they aren't dealt with in a timely manner. Due to a considerable reduction in face-to-face work by health and social care workers, many behavioural and psychological interventions cannot beconducted, making access to appropriate interventions more difficult.

SUPPORTING PEOPLE INFECTED WITH COVID-19

In many nations, the prevalence of the virus is not known because of a lack of planned and proactive testing for the virus. Infectious disease can have a devastating effect on elderly persons living in community residential facilities, as seen by the cases of elderly residents infected (Burcelinet al., 2015).As far as infection rates among people with ID are concerned, there is little evidence to go on. Infectious diseases need that support personnel modify their methods, but many feel that their health care system has failed to sufficiently protect them by providing personal protective equipment (PPE) and the expertise necessary to care for infected patients(Courtenay& Perera, 2020). In order to alleviate the strain on in-patient services, care workers are encouragedto learn new nursing skills and execute them in the community. People infected with the virus must be cared for using barrier nursing and infection control procedures. People with ID who are youngand healthy may not appreciate the need of sticking to infection control when they are being cared for. When staff members are away due to illness or the need to self-isolate, services may be affected. The WHO's (2020) recommendation that caregivers in the community have access to personal protective equipment has become a concern due to global shortages of equipment (Cooper, Smiley, Morrison, Williamson, & Allan, 2007).

.

The risk of harm from others

People with ID have a significant risk of damage from others, as illustrated by the Winterbourne View Hospital and Whorlton Hall scandals (Cooper et al., 2007). People who have been abusedor are at risk of being abused are protected by statutory systems. In light of the pandemic's surgein domestic violence in the general community, providers should be aware of an increased riskfor persons with ID(Burcelin et al., 2015).Clinicians may be unable to get a sense of a patient's safety as a result of changes in work practises to comply with physical separation and distant communication (Crawley et al., 2020; Yen et al., 2020) Doctors and other members of a person's social network may not be able to apply the traditional techniques of determining safety, and new approaches must be devised to protect them from damage. During the pandemic, it may be more difficult to conduct safeguarding investigations that rely on collecting information on allegations of abuse. Safeguarding interviews will increasingly be conducted via technology, and social distance as well as the use of PPE will be needed in situations where face-to-face contactis required.

SOCIAL IMPACTS OF THE PANDEMIC

While the pandemic's immediate effects on society are obvious, what about the long-term effectson people's health and well-being? However, it is not certain how the pandemic would influence the mental health of people with ID, who may perceive the social upheaval in a distinct way tothe general population. There are likely to be new ways of working for clinical professionals who care for persons with ID, which could lead to more efficient and simplified services. The new technology and processes will necessitate training for employees to guarantee that they are bothsuccessful and secure from data breaches.

ESSENTIAL STEPS FOR BETTER CARE

INCREASING VACCINATION

People with intellectual disabilities can be severely affected by vaccinations. Tennessee, whichwas the first state to include people with intellectual disabilities in its initial vaccination launch, saw an 80 percent decline in new COVID-19 infections among such individuals and caregivers from December 2020 to February 2021. Images portraying the vaccination procedure, rather than just words, should be used to educate persons with intellectual disabilities about the vaccines theyreceive. People with intellectual disabilities need to be educated about vaccinations and how tokeep them distracted, such as by providing a squeeze ball. Schedule appointments to minimise waiting time, which can be difficult for this more-sensitive demographic, and keep beneficiaries informed as to when they can depart. In the end, it all pays off. Jefferson Health immunised 50 adults with intellectual disabilities in six hours during a recent vaccination session in South Philadelphia. While quick vaccination of people with intellectual impairments is crucial during the epidemic, there is much more that can be done to improve their care in the future.

IMPROVING EDUCATION AND REDUCING BIAS

People with intellectual disabilities must be included in medical school curricula on a regular basis. It's important to address misconceptions about the sexuality of this demographic, for example, in an OB/GYN course. It is also recommended that students learn how to interview and assess people with intellectual disabilities using standardised patients, trained laypeople who act out medicalscenarios.

People with intellectual impairments can be a powerful source of information about what matters to them in health care, which can subsequently be shared with students and providers. People with intellectual disabilities should be given more opportunities at hospitals and doctors' offices in order to better understand and lessen their biases.

PROVIDING ACCOMMODATIONS AND APPROPRIATE SUPPORTS

A patient with an intellectual handicap may require assistance in communicating successfully, despite the requirement to limit visitors to prevent the spread of COVID-19. Long-term caretakers often have a better understanding of how to read a person's body language and how to makethem feel safe and secure.

For those who are very sensitive to loud noises, noise-cancelling headphones can help alleviate their discomfort.

Preparing these patients for the prospect of hospitalisation in advance is also helpful, so that theirhealth care wishes can be honoured. collaborating with one another and raising awareness

Diversity and equity goals in hospitals and health care systems need to include afocus on people with disabilities.

One of the first steps is to form advisory groups for people with intellectual disabilities who may discuss their health concerns and recommend solutions. There are educational opportunitiesavailable for patients who want to learn to advocate for themselves. These kinds of actions also serve to transform the culture of an institution by making this group of people more visible.

Allies in the health care field might advocate for more comprehensive insurance coverage forpeople with intellectual disabilities, for example. Providers must devote more time to meaningful communication and care coordination for these patients, and payers must cover that cost.

It's also critical to raise public awareness of the issue. Following the publication of our study on theadverse effects of the COVID-19 vaccination on people with intellectual disabilities, 11 statesdecided to include these individuals in their vaccine rollout priority groups.

PREVENTING DISCRIMINATION IN TREATMENT RATIONING

There is a pressing need to educate states and hospitals about federal disability rights statutes and their role in developing treatment rationing strategies. In order to ensure that people withdisabilities are treated in a nondiscriminatory manner, they need to be informed about their rights.The need for lawyers to address the rationing of ventilators, medications, and therapy for people with impairments

WORKFORCE SAFETY AND ADEQUACY

A lack of Personal Protective Equipment (PPE) for direct support workers has been reported by a number of organisations. The medical materials needed to safely quarantine people with impairments are not readily available, according to agencies.

ACCESS TO FOOD AND OTHER GROCERY

Items o Group homes and assisted living facilities are unable to procure enough food and materials for their clients and employees to eat three meals a day (e.g. food, including food for special diets, incontinence supplies, paper goods, supplemental nutrition products) O Family caregivers unable to pick up school meals from local authorities o Family caregivers unable toleave their houses in order to procure food and medication (e.g. gloves, hand sanitizer, toilet paper, disposable underwear, blue pads, adult diapers, paper goods, supplemental nutrition products, specialised nutrition products)

CONCLUSION

This year's COVID19 has had a significant impact on people all across the world. The focus is on those who will be most impacted by the pandemic. To be adequately shielded from the epidemic, people's identities must have been exposed to it firsthand. As a result of their intrinsic vulnerability to infection and the societal ramifications of the efforts taken to battle the epidemic, persons with an identity must be protected. Individuals with IDs and their caretakers must not beforgotten during a pandemic so that they can be prepared to handle similar situations in thefuture.

REFERENCES:

Burcelin, R., Courtney, M., & Amar, J. (2015). Gut microbiota and metabolic diseases: frompathogenesis to therapeutic perspective. In *Metabonomics and gut microbiota in nutrition and disease* (pp. 199-234): Springer.

Cooper, S.-A., Smiley, E., Morrison, J., Williamson, A., & Allan, L. (2007). Mental ill-health in adultswith intellectual disabilities: prevalence and associated factors. *The British journal of psychiatry, 190*(1), 27-35. doi:https://doi.org/10.1192/bjp.bp.106.022483

Courtenay, K., & Perera, B. (2020). COVID-19 and people with intellectual disability: impacts of apandemic. *Irish Journal of Psychological Medicine, 37*(3), 231-236. doi:https://doi.org/10.1017/ipm.2020.45

Crawley, E., Loades, M., Feder, G., Logan, S., Redwood, S., & Macleod, J. (2020). Wider collateraldamage to children in the UK because of the social distancing measures designed to reduce the impact of COVID-19 in adults. *BMJ Paediatrics Open, 4*(1). doi:https://doi.org/10.1136/bmjpo-2020-000701

Jm, V. B. (2010). Outbreak of pandemic virus (H1N1) 2009 in a residence for mentally disabledpersons in Balearic Island, Spain. *Revista espanola de salud publica, 84*(5), 665-670. doi:https://doi.org/10.1590/S1135-57272010000500017

Moghadas, S. M., Fitzpatrick, M. C., Sah, P., Pandey, A., Shoukat, A., Singer, B. H., & Galvani, A. P.(2020). The implications of silent transmission for the control of COVID-19 outbreaks. *Proceedings of the National Academy of Sciences, 117*(30), 17513-17515. doi:https://doi.org/10.1073/pnas.2008373117

Yen, M.-Y., Schwartz, J., Chen, S.-Y., King, C.-C., Yang, G.-Y., & Hsueh, P.-R. (2020). Interrupting COVID-19 transmission by implementing enhanced traffic control bundling: Implications for global prevention and control efforts. *Journal of Microbiology, Immunology and Infection, 53*(3), 377-380

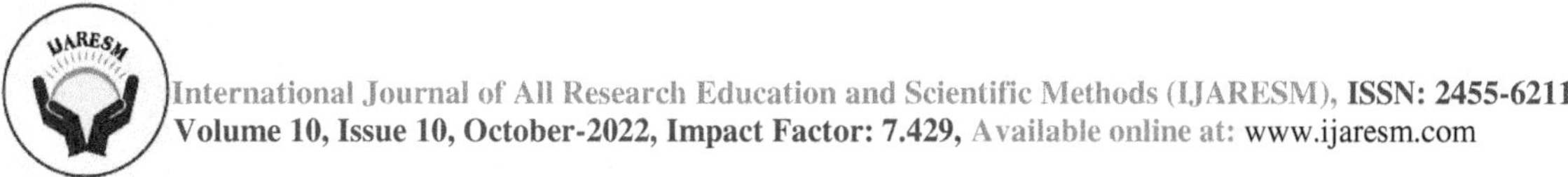
International Journal of All Research Education and Scientific Methods (IJARESM), ISSN: 2455-6211
Volume 10, Issue 10, October-2022, Impact Factor: 7.429, Available online at: www.ijaresm.com

"A Study to Assess the Knowledge, Attitude and Practice Regarding Covid-19 Management among Pregnant Women Attending Antenatal OPD at Sree Balaji Medical College and Hospital"

Dr. V. Hemavathy[1], Dr. Sathyalathasarathy[2], R. Sangeetha[3]

[1]Principal, Sree Balaji College of Nursing, Chrompet, Chennai
[2]HOD, Obstetrics and Gynecology Nursing Dept., Sree Balaji College of Nursing, Chrompet, Chennai
[3]MSc. Nursing, Sree Balaji College of Nursing, Chrompet, Chennai

****

ABSTRACT

Pandemics are large-scale outbreaks of infectious disease that can greatly increase morbidity and mortality over a wide geographic area and cause significant economic, social, and political disruption. The world has endured several notable pandemics, including the Black Death, Spanish flu, and human immunodeficiency virus/acquired immune deficiency syndrome (HIV/AIDS).On 31 December 2019, a cluster of cases of pneumonia of unknown cause, in the city of Wuhan, Hubei province in China, was reported to the World Health Organization. This novel coronavirus was named Coronavirus Disease 2019 (COVID-19) by WHO in February 2020.The virus is referred to as SARS-CoV-2 and the associated disease is COVID-19.Transmission of the virus is known to occur most often through close contact with an infected person (within 2 meters) or from contaminated surfaces.

Pregnant women do not appear more likely to contract the infection than the general population. However, pregnancy itself alters the body's immune system and response to viral infections in general, which can occasionally be related to more severe symptoms and this will be the same for COVID-19.Although higher maternal age, presence of comorbidities, and high body mass index have been considered as risk factors for developing severe COVID-19 in expecting mothers. Although higher maternal age, presence of comorbidities, and high body mass index have been considered as risk factors for developing severe COVID-19 in expecting mothers. There are case reports of preterm birth in women with COVID-19 and trans-placental transmission of COVID-19 has been recorded.

As COVID-19 is rapidly spreading, maternal management and fetal safety become a major concern, but there is scarce information of assessment and management of pregnant women infected with COVID-19, and the potential risk of vertical transmission is unclear. It has posed problem to both the antenatal women and maternity care workers. The care and management of pregnant women is an essential service to identify high-risk mothers and also to have good pregnancy outcome for both mother and baby.

Keywords: Coronavirus disease 2019, Severe acute respiratory syndrome coronavirus 2 (SARS-CoV-2). COVID-19 in pregnancy, Pregnancy outcome, vertical transmission, vaccination.

OBJECTIVES

1. To assess the pre -test level of knowledge, attitude and practice regarding covid-19 management among pregnant women attending antenatal OPD at Sree Balaji Hospital and Medical College.
2. To assess the post- test level of knowledge, attitude and practice regarding covid-19 management among pregnant women attending antenatal OPD at Sree Balaji Medical College and hospital.
3. To evaluate the effectiveness of educational intervention package regarding Covid-19 management among pregnant women attending antenatal OPD at Sree Balaji Medical College and Hospital.
4. To associate with Post -test level of knowledge, attitude & practice score regarding Covid-19 management with selected demographic variables among pregnant women attending antenatal OPD at Sree Balaji Medical College and Hospital.

RESEARCH DESIGN

This study was conducted on a convenient sample of 60 pregnant women at Sree Balaji Medical College and Hospital, Chennai. The pregnant women were between the age group of 24 to 40 years.

NULL HYPOTHESIS

1. **NH 1** - There is no significant association between pre -test and post- test level of knowledge, attitude & practice regarding Covid-19 management among pregnant women attending antenatal OPD at Sree Balaji Medical College and Hospital.

2. **NH 2** - There is no significant association between Post- test level of knowledge, attitude & practice score regarding Covid-19 management with selected demographic variables of pregnant women attending antenatal OPD at Sree Balaji Medical College and Hospital.

RESULT

In the pre-test out of 60 pregnant women, 26 (43.3 %) of pregnant women were having inadequate knowledge, 28 (46.6 %) of pregnant women were having moderately adequate knowledge, 6 (10%) of pregnant women were having adequate knowledge. Overall the pre-test mean score was 48.5 with standard deviation of 21.7 . In the pre-test the data analysed showed that out of 60 pregnant women 13(21.6 %) of pregnant women were having unfavorable attitude, 21 (35 %) of pregnant women were having neutral attitude, 26 (43%) of pregnant women were having favorable attitude. Overall the pre-test attitude mean score was 82.8 with the standard deviation of 9.4. In the practice assessment of pregnant women regarding Covi-19 management, among 60 women 0(0 %) of pregnant women were having rarely practice, 13 (21.6 %) of pregnant women were having sometimes practice, 47 (78.3%) of pregnant women mostly practice. The overall practice mean score for was 86.6 and standard deviation is 3.2.

In the post-test out of 60 pregnant women, 10 (16.6 %) of pregnant women were having moderately adequate knowledge, 50 (83.3%) of pregnant women were having adequate knowledge. Overall the post-test attitude mean score was 82.8 with the standard deviation of 9.4. The result of post-test attitude assessment among pregnant women shows 13 (21.6 %) of pregnant women were having neutral attitude, 47 (78.3%) of pregnant women were having favorable attitude. Overall post-test attitude mean score was 81.6 with standard deviation 10.4. The result of data analysis of post-test practice assessment regarding Covid-19 management among pregnant women shows 0(0 %) of pregnant women rarely practice, 0 (0 %) of pregnant women sometimes practice, 60 (100%) of pregnant women mostly practice.

CONCLUSION

This chapter has brought out various implications of the study and has also provided suggestion for future studies. The constant encouragement and direction of the guide, co-operation and interest of the subjects to participate in the study had contributed to the fruitful and successful completion of the study. This study has shown that the educational intervention package is an effective strategy in improving the knowledge, attitude and practice of pregnant women regarding Covid-19 management. The pre-test mean value is 48.5 and standard deviation is 21.7. Post-test mean value is 82.8 and standard deviation is 9.4. The paired 't' value is 25.3 which is statistically significant at $p < 0.001$. Based on the analyzed data, it was felt that there is improvement in the post-test level of knowledge in experimental group. Hence the present study improved that the educational intervention package among pregnant women regarding Covid-19 management was effective.

REFERENCES

[1] https://onlinelibrary.wiley.com/doi/10.1002/jmv.27423
[2] https://obgyn.onlinelibrary.wiley.com/doi/10.1111/ajo.13204
[3] https://www.nature.com/articles/s41467-021-27745-z#Sec11
[4] https://www.jogi.co.in/storage/files/impact_of_the_coronavirus_infection_in_pregnancy_a_preliminary_study_of_141_patients-1.pdf
[5] https://www.sciencedirect.com/science/article/pii/S221339842100172X
[6] https://www.nature.com/articles/s41577-022-00703-6
[7] https://www.cdc.gov/coronavirus/2019-ncov/need-extra-precautions/pregnant-people.html

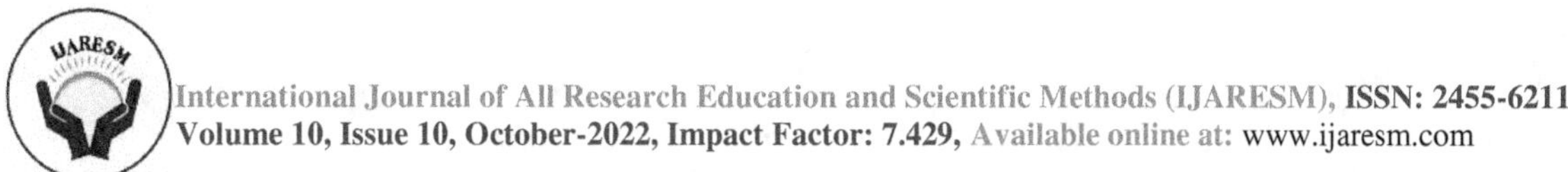
International Journal of All Research Education and Scientific Methods (IJARESM), ISSN: 2455-6211
Volume 10, Issue 10, October-2022, Impact Factor: 7.429, Available online at: www.ijaresm.com

"Effectiveness of Structured Teaching Programme on Knowledge andAttitude Regarding Post Covid Symptoms Management Among Frontline Workers (Nurses) At Selected Hospital In Chennai"

Dr. V. Hemavathy[1], Prof. Girija Baskaran[2], J. Regina Margret Vimala[3]

[1]Principal, Sree Balaji College Of Nursing, Chennai
[2]HOD, Dept. Of Medical Surgical Nursing, Sree Balaji College of Nursing, Chennai
[3]M. Sc (N), II Year, Sree Balaji College of Nursing, Chennai

****

INTRODUCTION

Severe acute respiratory syndrome coronavirus 2 (SARS-CoV-2) is the pathogen responsible for the coronavirusdisease 2019 (COVID-19) pandemic, which has resulted in global healthcare crises and strained health resources.Thepublic health impact of the SARS-CoV-2 pandemic is beyond everybody's imagination. This pandemic has affectedmore than 210 countries and a majority of these countries are still under some infection control measures, including quarantine, lockdown, and recommended or mandatory general facemask use, and social distancing in public areas Most people with COVID-19 get better within weeks of illness, whereas some patients experience new, recurring orongoing symptoms related to COVID-19 several weeks after the acute phase of infection The U.S. Centre for DiseaseControl and Prevention (CDC) recommends using the umbrella term "post-COVID conditions" for a wide range ofsigns and symptoms that occur four or more weeks after acute COVID-19 infection. Standardized case definitions are still being developed. In general, post-COVID conditions are characterized by a lack of return to a usual state of healthfollowing acute COVID-19 infection

Post-COVID conditions are a wide range of new, returning, or ongoing health problems people can experience **four or more weeks** after first being infected with the virus that causes COVID-19. Post-COVID conditions are referred to by a wide range of names, including "long COVID," "post-COVID syndrome," "post-acute COVID-19 syndrome," as well as the research term **"post-acute sequelae of SARS-CoV-2 infection" (PASC).** Among the lay public, the phrase "long-haulers" is also used

Even people who did not have COVID-19 symptoms in the days or weeks after they were infected can have post- COVID conditions. These conditions can present as different types and combinations of health problems for different lengths of time. As we are travelling in the second year of pandemic, patients with ongoing symptoms after recovery from COVID-19 are increasingly recognized as a growing population in need of attention.

OBJECTIVES :

1. To assess the pre test level of knowledge and attitude regarding post covid symptoms management amongfrontline workers (NURSES) in Sree Balaji Medical College and Hospital.
2. To assess the post test level of knowledge and attitude regarding post covid symptoms management amongfrontline workers (NURSES) in Sree Balaji Medical College and Hospital.
3. To compare the pre test and post test level of knowledge and attitude regarding post covid symptomsmanagement among the frontline workers (NURSES)
4. To associate the post test level of knowledge regarding post covid symptoms management among frontlineworkers (NURSES) with their selected demographic variables

METHODOLOGY

The quantitative research approach and one group pre test – post test design (pre experimental design) was used for the study. Non probability convenient sampling technique was used to select the sample for the study. A sample size of60 staff nurses was selected for this study. The study was conducted at Sree Balaji Medical College and Hospital ,Chrompet, Chennai . A structured questionnaire was developed based on the objectives of the study after reviewing related literature. The questionnaire consists of two parts. Part – I includes demographic variables and part – II consists of sections of questions based on covid and post covid symptom and management. Part – III involves Attitude based statements based on (Likert scale).

RESULTS

The study findings reveal that in this study, there were 60 (100%) frontline workers (NURSES) who participated. Among the participants There were 37 (61.60%) nurses in the age group between 21-30 years, 18 (30%) of nurses in the age group between 31-40 years and 5(8.30%) of nurses in the age group between 41-50 years.

Among the samples 8 (13.30%) of them were Male nurses and 42 (70%) were Female nurses.

With regard to religion out of 60 nurses, 40 (66.6%) were Hindus, 15 (25%) were Christians, and 5 (8.30%) were Muslims.

Out of 60 nurses, based on their educational status 22 (36.6%) nurses were general nursing midwifery qualified and 38 (63.3%) were graduates in nursing.

Based upon the experience, 37 (61.6%) nurses had experience within 1-2 years, 15 (25%) nurses had experience within3-5 years, and 5 (8.3%) nurses had experience above 5 years.

Regarding the areas of experience 43 (71.6%) nurses had worked only in wards, 10 (16.6%) nurses had worked only in intensive care units, 5(8.3%) of nurses had work experience in casualty and 2 (3.3%) of nurses had experience working in covid wards and ICU.

Next based upon the family history of covid – 19 , 28 (46.6%) nurses had members in their family with covid affected and 32 (53.3%) nurses had no family members affected with covid.

On seeing the history of covid vaccination 53 (88.3%) of nurses had been vaccinated and 7 (11.6%) was not vaccinated.

In pre test analysis majority of the frontline workers – nurses 56 (93.3%) have inadequate knowledge, 4 (6.60%) nurses had moderate knowledge and none fell under the category of adequate knowledge.

This clearly depicts knowledge on post covid and symptoms management among the nurses was very much lacking and it definitely had an impact in their pre test attitude assessment levels which were frontline workers – nurses 48 (80%) have inadequate attitude, and 12 (20%) nurses had moderate level of attitude and none fell under the category of adequate attitude.

Following the intervention of the structured teaching programme on post covid symptoms management, the post test analysis, 55 (91.6%) nurses gained adequate knowledge and 5 (8.30%) nurses had gained moderate knowledge and none fell under the category of inadequate knowledge and definitely impacted on their post test attitude levels which showed the majority of the frontline workers – nurses have gained adequate attitude ie 52 (80.6%) and 8 (13.3%) nurses had developed moderate level of attitude and none fell under the category of inadequate attitude.

The pre test mean score of knowledge among the nurses was 17.3 with standard deviation 8.8 and the post test mean score was 82.1 with standard deviation 9.7 the obtained paired "t" value was 54.6 which reveals that there was statistically highly significant difference between the pre test and post test .

Similarly thepre test mean score of attitude shows 22.0 with standard deviation of 14.1 and the post test mean score of attitude showed 80.3 with standard deviation of 12.0.

The obtained paired "t" value was 39.3 which reveals that there was statistically highly significant difference between the pre test and post test levels of knowledge and attitude from the study. Hence there is a significant differencebetween the pre and post level scores indicating that the structured teaching intervention was effective.

All the demographic variables had no association with the post test level of knowledge.

CONCLUSION

The results of the study shows that the structured reaching programme was effective in enhancing the knowledge and attitude of post covid symptoms management among nurses. Furthermore recognizing and upgrading the changing and added professional roles and responsibilities of the nurses will take them to a farther milestone in enabling them in tackling future pandemics.

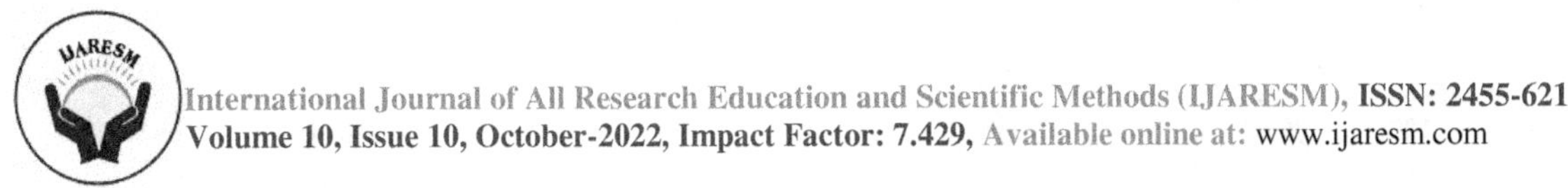
International Journal of All Research Education and Scientific Methods (IJARESM), ISSN: 2455-6211
Volume 10, Issue 10, October-2022, Impact Factor: 7.429, Available online at: www.ijaresm.com

A Study to Assess the Effectiveness of the Self Instructional Module on Awareness and Practice of Covid-19 Precautionary Measures among Rural Adults (20-50 Years) At Padappai

Dr. V. Hemavathy[1], Mrs. Vasanthakohila[2], Mrs. R. Dhivya[3]

[1]Principal, Sree Balaji College of Nursing
[2]HOD, Professor, Sree Balaji College of Nursing
[3]M.SC (N) IInd Year Student Sree Balaji College of Nursing

****

INTRODUCTION

According to the World Health Organization (WHO), viral diseases continue to emerge and represent a serious issue to public health. In the last twenty years, several viral epidemics such as the severe acute respiratory syndrome coronavirus (SARS- CoV) from 2002 to 2003, and H1N1 influenza in 2009, have been recorded. Most recently, the Middle East respiratory syndrome coronavirus (MERS-CoV) was first identified in Saudi Arabia in 2012 and now the new Coronavirus disease 2019 (COVID-19) has plagued the world. COVID-19 is an emerging respiratory disease caused by the highly contagious novel coronavirus (SARS-CoV 2) and was first detected in December 2019 in Wuhan, China . This new virus has quickly spread globally afflicting 215 countries. As of June 13th, 2020, over 7.8 million cases and 430,000 deaths have been reported globally A novel β-coronavirus designated as severe acute respiratory syndrome coronavirus−2 (SARS-CoV2) was identified as the causative agent of coronavirus disease 2019 (COVID-19). The first COVID-19 outbrea+k was reported in December 2019 in Wuhan, China. The rapid spread of the virus led the World Health Organization (WHO) to declare a Public Health Emergency of International Concern in January 2020 and a pandemic in March 2020. The various modes of transmission of COVID- 19 from human-to-human include contact via aerosols and droplets from infected individuals through coughing, sneezing or talking as well as fomites or contaminated surfaces. The risk of community transmission from asymptomatic carriers also contributes to the burden of disease. Although multiple vaccines are now available, their long-term efficacy is unknown, they may not beeffective against mutant strainsand are experiencing a high degree of hesitancy. Thus, the application of precautionary measures remains important to minimize pandemic spread and reduce mortality rate. There are a variety of practices that play an important role in controlling infection such as washing hands, wearing face masks, use of mouthwash, social distancing (stay at home) and isolating confirmed cases. These measures are Importa.nt for all members of the community.

Objectives Of The Study

- To assess the pretest level of knowledge regarding on awareness and practice of covid-19 precautionary measures among rural adults at padappai.
- To assess the post test level of knowledge regarding on awareness and practice of covid-19 precautionarymeasures among rural adults at padappai.
- To evaluate the effectiveness of the self instructional module on awareness and practice of covid-19 precautionary measures among rural adults at padappai.
- To associate the post test knowledge score with selected demographic variables among rural adults at padappai.

METHODOLOGY

The quantitative research approach and one group pre test - post test design was used for the study. Convenient sampling technique was used to select the sample for the study. A sample size of 100 rural adults were selected for this study. The study was conducted in padappai, chennai. The structured interview questionnaire was developed based on the objectives of the study after reviewing the literature. The questionnaire consists of two parts . part I includes demographic variables and part II consists of 30 closed ended questions regarding covid -19 precautionary measures.

RESULTS

The level of knowledge of rural adults in the pre test was 3(3%) of them had inadequate knowledge , 58(58%) of them had moderate level of knowledge and 39(39%) of them had adequate level of knowledge on covid -19 precautionary measures. In the post test among the 100 rural adults 0(0%) of them had inadequateknowledge , 4(4%) of them had moderate level of knowledge and 96(96%) of them had adequate level of knowledge on covid -19 precautionary

measures. This shows that the self instructional module was effective. Over all the paired 't' test score was 21.9 which is highly significant at p<0.001. The variables showed that there was no significant association between the selected demographic variables and the post test level of knowledge of rural adults on covid-19 precautionary measures.

CONCLUSION

The study showed that there was significant improvement at p<0.001 in the post test knowledge. It also shows that there is no association between the selected demographic variables and the post test knowledge level. Thus the self instructional module imparted to the rural adults on covid-19 precautionary measures had an effect on their knowledge and had a great potential for accelerating the awareness among rural adults.

BIBLIOGRAPHY

[1] Naif K Binsaleh Awareness and Practice of COVID-19 Precautionary Measures Among Healthcare Professionals in Saudi Arabia . 2021 Jun 22.

[2] Francis Enenche Ejeh Knowledge, attitude, and practice among healthcare workers towards COVID-19 outbreakin Nigeria pub 2020 Nov 18.

[3] Rothan H.A., Byrareddy S.N. The epidemiology and pathogenesis of coronavirus disease (COVID-19) outbreak. J. Autoimmun. 2020

[4] Andersen K.G., Rambaut A., Lipkin W.I., Holmes E.C., Garry R.F. The proximal origin of SARS-CoV-2. Nat. Med. 2020

[5] Kannan S., Shaik Syed Ali P., Sheeza A., Hemalatha K. COVID-19 (Novel Coronavirus 2019) - recent trends.Eur. Rev. Med. Pharmacol. Sci. 2020;24:2006–2011

International Journal of All Research Education and Scientific Methods (IJARESM), ISSN: 2455-6211
Volume 10, Issue 10, October-2022, Impact Factor: 7.429, Available online at: www.ijaresm.com

A Study to Assess the Effectiveness of Structured Teaching Programme on the Knowledge and Attitude of the Long Standing Practice Contributing To Risk of Varicosity among Guards at Selected Hospital

Dr. V. Hemavathy[1], Mrs. Girija Bhaskaran[2], Miss. Pooja. R. Bhatt[3]

[1]Principal, Sree Balaji College Of Nursing
[2]Professor, H.O.D Of Medical Surgical Nursing, Sree Balaji College of Nursing
[3]M.SC (N)2ND Year Student of Sree Balaji College of Nursing

****

INTRODUCTION

Varicose veins are one of the chief preventable diseases which are associated with veins. It is a serious disease, which poses threat to life of patient when effective and efficient measures arenot taken. Modern world a lot of occupations and professions have designed up where people are required to either continuously stand for a long time or made to sit hanging down for a considerabletime. The work environment constitutes an important part of man's total environment. Health to a large extent is affected by work conditions. Occupational environment too plays a major role on thehealth of the exposed. The health hazards get more severe when the duration of exposure increases.1Millions of workers spend themajority of the working day on their feet and many hours in static positions. Prolonged standing can lead to tiredness, loss of concentration and increased health riskssuch as the swelling of feet and legs, feet and joint damage, varicose veins, heart and circulatory disorders and lower back problems. Severe varicose veins can have an impact on the lives ofthe people who work on their feet especially the teachers, nursing staffs, flight attendants, dental staff, traffic and bar workers, postal workers, construction workers and bank staff. The reason is the samefor the security guards, who are as apart of their profession need to stand for prolonged periods, placing them at the highest risk of developing varicose veins.

The term varicose derives from the Latin 'varix', which means twisted. A varicose veinis usually tortuous and dilated. Under normal circumstances, blood collected from superficial venouscapillaries is directed upward and inward via one- way valves into superficial veins. These, in turn, drain via perforator veins, which pass through muscle fascia into deeperveins buried under the fascia.Leakage in a valve caused retrograde flow back into the vein. Unlike deep veins which are thick-walled and confined by fascia, superficial veins cannot withstand high pressure and eventually becomedilated andtortuous.

OBJECTIVES:

1. To assess the pre-test level of knowledge and attitude of the longstanding practice contributing to risk of varicosity among security guards

2. To assess the post-test level of knowledge and attitude of the longstanding practice contributing to risk of varicosity among security guards

3. To compare the pre-test and post-test level of knowledge and attitude of the longstanding practice contributing torisk of varicosity among security guards.

4. To associate the post- test level of knowledge of the longstanding practice contributing to risk of varicosity among security guards with selected demographic variables.

METHODOLOGY

The research design used for the present study was pre experimental one group pretest, posttest design. The research setting was Sree Balaji Medical College and Hospital , Chennai-44. Sample size was 60 students selected by non- probability convenient sampling technique.

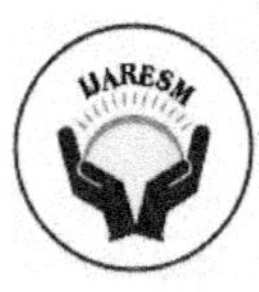

RESULT

In pre-test majority of the security guards 60(100%) have inadequate knowledge. No one has moderately adequate or adequate knowledge regarding prevention of varicose vein. It denotes that the security guards have very less or no knowledge about prevention of varicose vein. In post-test 9(15) gained moderately adequate knowledge, 16(26.66) gained adequate knowledge, 35(58.33) had inadequate knowledge. Also the pre-test mean and standard deviation was

and 18.7. Thepost-test mean and standard deviation was 65.2 and 22.6. The paired't' test value was 16.3, which reveals there was statistically highly significant at p<0.001. Therefore, the structured teaching program regarding prevention of varicose vein among the security gaurds was found to be effective.

All the demographic variables had no significant association with the post-test level of knowledge, except religion is significant association.

CONCLUSION

The Results of the study shows that the structured teaching program was effective in improved their knowledge level regarding prevention of varicose vein. Furthermore with changes in lifestyle many non-communicable diseases like coronary artery diseases, diabetes are on trends so, there are higher chances for people getting varicose vein. Thus, the prevention of varicose vein programme can be implemented in colleges for the teachers as well as the students in order to create awareness and lead health life.

BIBLIOGRAPHY

[1] Brunner and Suddharth (2014),textbook of medical surgical nursing ,volume I, 13th edition Philapelphia: Wolter Kluwer publications
[2] Neil R.Standing problem ,Hazards Magazine (online) 2005 Aug 10
[3] Harrison ,Principal of Internal medicine ,12th edition ,Mc Graw hill ,page number 1024-1025.

International Journal of All Research Education and Scientific Methods (IJARESM), ISSN: 2455-6211
Volume 10, Issue 10, October-2022, Impact Factor: 7.429, Available online at: www.ijaresm.com

"A Study To Assess The Effectiveness of Instructional Media on Stress Among Late Adolescence During Covid-19 Pandemic At Sree Balaji College of Nursing, Chrompet"

Dr. V. Hemavathy[1], Miss. S. Lavanya[2]

[1]Principal, Sree Balaji College Of Nursing
[2]M.SC (N) 2nd Year Student Of Sree Balaji College Of Nursing

INTRODUCTION

In December 2019, a cluster of atypical cases of pneumonia was reported in Wuhan, China, which was later designated as Corona virus disease (COVID-19) by the World Health Organization (WHO) on 11 Feb 2020. The causative virus, SARS-CoV-2, was identified as a novel strain of corona viruses that shares 79% genetic similarity with SARS-Covid from the 2003 SARS outbreak. On 11 Mar 2020, the WHO declared the outbreak a global pandemic, COVID-19 pandemic has affected all levels of the education system around the world (in 192 countries) have either temporarily closed or implemented localized closures affecting about 1.7 billion student population worldwide. Many universities around the world either postponed orcancelled all campus activities to minimize gatherings and hence decrease the transmission of the virus. However, these measures lead to higher economical, medical, and social implications. Students have reported higher rates of stress, anxiety and depression in online classes compared to offline classes.

This contagious virus has not only raised concerns over general public health, but has also caused a number of psychological and mental disorders. According to our analysis, it can be concluded that the COVID-19 pandemiccan affect mental health in individuals and different communities. Therefore, in the current crisis, it is vital to identify individuals prone to stress from different groups and at different layers of populations, so that with appropriate instructional media regarding stress, the adolescent's mental health is preserved and improved.It is natural to feel stress, anxiety, grief, and worry during the COVID-19 pandemic.

Keywords: COVID-19, global pandemic, mental health .

OBJECTIVES OF THE STUDY

- To assess the pre- test level of stress among late adolescence during covid-19 pandemic.
- To assess the post-test level stress among late adolescence during covid-19 pandemic.
- To assess the effectiveness of instructional media on stress among late adolescenceduring covid-19 pandemicby comparing the score of pre-test &post level.
- To associate the post-test level of stress with selected demographic variable.

METHODOLOGY

The research design used in the present study was pre-experiment one group pre-test and post-test design. The research setting was Sree Balaji College of Nursing, Chrompet. Sample size was 60 late adolescences selected by non- probability convenient sampling technique.

RESULT

In the pre-test among 60 samples of nursing students, 18(3%) of them had low stress in pre- test, 32(53.3%) of them had moderate stress, 10(16.70%) had high stress level. It denotes thatmost of them had experienced stress during covid-19 pandemic. In post-test among 60 samplesof nursing students 41(68.33%) of them had low stress, 19(31.66%) of them had moderate stress and 0(0%) of them had high stress. Also, in pre-test mean and standard deviation was 18.0 and 9.2. The post-test means and standard deviation was 10.4 and 6.6. the paired 't' valuewas 11.3, which reveal there was statistically significant at p<0.001. Therefore, the instructional media on stress during covid-19 pandemic among late adolescence was found to be effective.

All the demographical variables had no association with post-level of knowledge.

CONCLUSION

The result of the study shows that the instructional media was effective in improvement of their knowledge level regarding covid-19 pandemic stress and how to handle it. Further more Stress has an advantages and disadvantages. If people will handle stress effectively this can provide a lot of advantages to people. But if people will not handle stress effectively this maylead a lot problem to people. Stress is a common problem in modern life. Managing stress at work means learning to manage situations differently but it also means learning how to manage oneself, knowing one's resources and making better use of one's personal abilities.

REFERENCES

[1] Ahuja Niraj (2002) A Short text book of psychiatry 1st edition ,New Delhi, Jaypeepublishers.
[2] BT Basavanthappa (2000) Nursing research 2nd edition ,Bangalore, Jaypee publishers.
[3] https://eujournal.org.
[4] https://scholar.google.co.in.

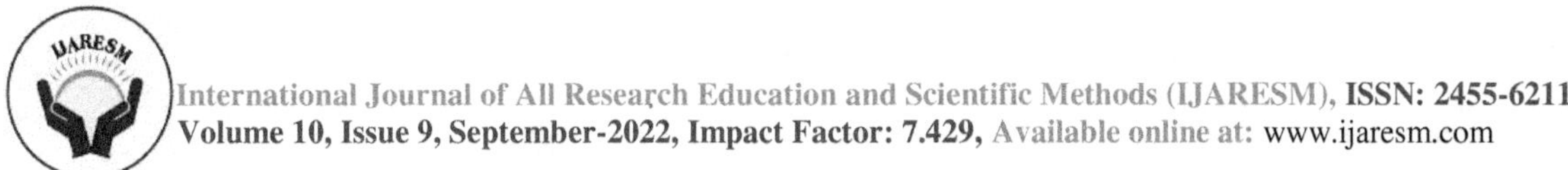
International Journal of All Research Education and Scientific Methods (IJARESM), ISSN: 2455-6211
Volume 10, Issue 9, September-2022, Impact Factor: 7.429, Available online at: www.ijaresm.com

Respiratory Syncytial Virus

Dr. V. Hemavathy[1], Mrs. Vasanthakohila[2], Mrs. R. Dhivya[3]

[1]Principal, Sree Balaji College of Nursing
[2]HOD, Professor, Sree Balaji College of Nursing
[3]M.SC (N) IInd Year Student Sree Balaji College of Nursing

****

ABSTRACT

Respiratory syncytial virus (RSV) is the most common single cause of respiratory hospitalization of infants and is the second largest cause of lower respiratory infection mortality worldwide. In adults, RSV is an under-recognised cause of deterioration in health, particularly in frail elderly persons. Infection rates typically rise in late autumn and early winter causing bronchiolitis in infants, common colds in adults and insidious respiratory illness in the elderly. Virus detection methods optimised for use in children have low detection rate in adults, highlighting the need for better diagnostic tests. There are many vaccines under development, mostly based on the surface glycoprotein F which exists in two conformations (prefusion and postfusion). Much of the neutralising antibody appears to be to the prefusion form. Vaccines being developed include live attenuated, subunit, particle based and live vectored agents. Different vaccine strategies may be appropriate for different target populations: at-risk infants, school-age children, adult caregivers and the elderly. Antiviral drugs are in clinical trial and may find a place in disease management. RSV disease is one of the major remaining common tractable challenges in infectious diseases and the era of vaccines and antivirals for RSV is on the near horizon.

Keywords: copd exacerbations; innate immunity; paediatric lung disaese; viral infection.

INTRODUCTION

Respiratory syncytial virus (RSV) is a common respiratory virus. It affects the lungs and its bronchioles (smaller passageways that carry air to the lung). RSV is one of the most common causes of childhood illness, infecting most children by two years of age. RSV can also infect adults.

Most healthy children and older adults who get RSV will get a mild case with cold-like symptoms. Only self-care or "comfort care" is usually needed.

Severe infection with RSV can lead to pneumonia (an infection in the lungs) and bronchiolitis (inflammation of the small airways in the lungs) and may require hospital care. People at greatest risk of severe infection are the very young (those less than six months old), those over the age of 65 and those of any age who have heart or lung conditions or a weakened immune system. RSV can also make existing heart and lung problems worse.

DEFINITION

A paramyxovirus which causes disease of the respiratory tract. It is a major cause of bronchiolitis and pneumonia in young children, and may be a contributing factor in cot death.

CAUSES

Respiratory syncytial virus enters the body through the eyes, nose or mouth. It spreads easily through the air on infected respiratory droplets. You or your child can become infected if someone with RSV coughs or sneezes near you. The virus also passes to others through direct contact, such as shaking hands.

The virus can live for hours on hard objects such as countertops, crib rails and toys. Touch your mouth, nose or eyes after touching a contaminated object and you're likely to pick up the virus.

SIGNS AND SYMPTOMS

Common symptoms of RSV in infants include:

- Runny nose.
- Decrease in appetite.
- Sneezing and coughing.
- Fever (temperature above 100 degrees Fahrenheit). Fever may not always be present.

Symptoms in the youngest infants include:

- Fussiness/irritability.
- Decreased activity/more tired than usual.
- Decreased appetite.
- Pauses in breathing.

Symptoms of severe RSV in infants include:

- Short, shallow and rapid breathing.
- Flaring (spreading out) of nostrils with every breath.
- Belly breathing (look for a "caving in" of the chest in the form of an upside-down "V" starting under the neck).
- Bluish coloring of lips, mouth and fingernails.
- Wheezing (This can be a sign of pneumonia or bronchiolitis.)
- Poor appetite.

DIAGNOSTIC EVALUATION

- Child's medical history and ask about symptoms.
- The physical exam will include listening to your or your child's lungs and checking oxygen level in a simple finger monitoring test (pulse oximetry).
- They may order blood testing to check for signs of infection (such as a higher than normal white blood cell count)or take a nose swab to test for viruses.

If more severe illness is suspected, your healthcare provider will order imaging tests (X-rays, CT scan) to check your or your child's lungs.

MANAGEMENT

If you or your child has mild symptoms, prescription treatment is usually not needed. RSV goes away on its own in oneto two weeks. Antibiotics are not used to treat viral infections, including those caused by RSV. (Antibiotics may be prescribed, however, if testing shows you or your child has bacterial pneumonia or other infection.)

Some young children who develop bronchiolitis may have to be hospitalized to receive oxygen treatment. If your child is unable to drink because of rapid breathing, he or she may need to receive intravenous fluids to stay hydrated. On rare occasions, infected babies will need a respirator to help them breathe. Only about 3% of children with RSV require a hospital stay. Most children are able to go home from the hospital in two or three days.

If you are an older adult and especially if you have a weakened immune system, you may need to be hospitalized if the RSV is severe. While in the hospital, you may receive oxygen or be put on a breathing machine (ventilator) to help your breathe or receive IV fluids to help with dehydration.

PREVENTION

- Wash your hands often. Wash for 20 seconds. If soap and water are not available, use an alcohol-based hand sanitizer that contains at least 60% alcohol. (Alcohol-based rubs work well for young children who don't have the coordination or attention span for proper hand washing technique.)
- Avoid touching your eyes, nose and mouth to prevent the spread of viruses from your hands.
- Cover your mouth and nose with a tissue when sneezing and coughing or sneeze and cough into your elbow. Throw the tissue in the trash. Wash your hands afterward. Never cough or sneeze into your hands!
- Avoid close contact (within 6 feet) with those who have known RSV, coughs, colds or are sick. Stay home ifyou are sick.

- Don't share cups, toys or bottles, or any objects. Viruses may be able to live on such surfaces for hours (andbe transmitted to your hands).
- If you are prone to sickness or have a weakened immune system, stay away from large crowds of people.
- Clean frequently used surfaces (such as doorknobs and counter tops) with a virus-killing disinfectant.

Additional tips for children:

- Keeping your children home from day care when they or other children become ill.
- If you have a child at high risk of developing severe RSV, try to limit time at child care centers or gatheringsof large number of children during the RSV season.
- Wash toys frequently.

CONCLUSION

RSV is an important agent causing lower obstructive airway disease (34.3% of all patients). There are no specific symptoms that can be used for diagnosing RSV infection. In order to prevent other patients on the ward from contracting nosocomial RSV infection and in the light of therapeutic options, one should test newly admitted patients presenting with symptoms of an obstructive airway disease for RSV antigen. On a ward with high-risk patients, we would recommend the use of an RSV test for all new patients.

REFERENCES

[1] https://pubmed.ncbi.nlm.nih.gov/10697789/#:~:text=Conclusion%3A%20RSV%20is%20an%20important,used%20for%20diagnosing%20RSV%20infection.
[2] https://www.ncbi.nlm.nih.gov/pmc/articles/PMC3461981/
[3] https://www.mayoclinic.org/diseases-conditions/respiratory-syncytial-virus/symptoms-causes/syc-20353098
[4] https://medlineplus.gov/ency/article/001564.htm

International Journal of All Research Education and Scientific Methods (IJARESM), **ISSN: 2455-6211**
Volume 10, Issue 9, September-2022, Impact Factor: 7.429, Available online at: www.ijaresm.com

Insomnia

Dr. V. Hemavathy[1], Miss. M. Ranjini[2]

[1]Principal, Sree Balaji College of Nursing
[2]M.SC (N) 2nd Year Student of Sree Balaji College of Nursing

****

ABSTRACT

Insomnia is the most common type of sleep disorder in the family medicine population. It is defined as a persistent difficulty initiating or maintaining sleep, or a report of nonrestorative sleep, accompanied by related daytime impairment. Insomnia is a significant public health problem because of its high prevalence and management challenges. There is increasing evidence of a strong association between insomnia and various medical and psychiatric comorbidities. Diagnosis of insomnia and treatment planning rely on a thorough sleep history to address contributing and precipitating factors as well as maladaptive behaviors resulting in poor sleep. Using a sleep diary or sleep log is more accurate than patient recall to determine sleep patterns. A sleep study is not routinely indicated for evaluation of insomnia. Cognitive behavioral therapy for insomnia (CBT-I) is the mainstay of treatment and is asafe and effective approach.

Key words: sleep disorder, maladaptive behavior, cognitive behavioral therapy

INTRODUCTION

Insomnia is a common sleep complaint that occurs when you have one or more of theseproblems:

- Havingahardtime in initiating sleep.
- Struggling to maintain sleep, wakingupfrequentlyduringthenight.
- Tendency towakeuptooearlyandareunabletogobacktosleep.

These symptoms of insomnia can be caused by a variety of biological, psychological and social factors. They most often result in an inadequate amount of sleep, even though the sufferer has the opportunity to get a full night of sleep

Prevalence:

Insomnia symptoms occur in approximately 33% to 50% of the adult population while Chronic Insomnia disorder that is associated with distress or impairment is estimated at 10% to 15%.

Types of insomnia:

Chronic insomnia
It is defined to occur at least 3 nights per week for at least 3 months. It may last for years or even decades.

Short-term insomnia (or acute insomnia)
It lasts less than 3 months with an unspecified frequency.

Subtypes

Psychophysiological insomnia: heightened arousal with excessive worry and focus on sleep.
Idiopathic insomnia: longstanding and genetically based, often beginning in infancy or childhood.
Paradoxical insomnia: sleep state misperception resulting in mistaken belief that sleep has not occurred.

Inadequate sleep hygiene: habits that disturb sleep including naps, caffeine intake, a variable sleepschedule, and using the bedroom for non-sleep activities. sleep lightly or briefly, especially during the day.

Behavioral insomnia of childhood: usually either sleep-onset type in infants or limit-setting type intoddlers. A toddler is a child 12 to 36 months old Insomnia due to a mental disorder: most often to anxiety or depression.

Insomnia due to a medical condition: most often chronic pain or sleep apnea.

Insomnia due to drug or substance: may be due to intoxication or withdrawal from over-the-counter, prescription, or illicit substances.

Risk Groups

- A high rate of insomnia is seen in middle-aged and older adults. Although your individual sleep need does not change as you age, physical problems can make it more difficult to sleep well.
- Women are more likely than men to develop insomnia.
- People who have a medical or psychiatric illness, including depression, are at risk for insomnia.
- People who use medications may experience insomnia as a side-effect.

Effects

- Fatigue
- Moodiness
- Irritability or anger
- Daytime sleepiness
- Anxiety about sleep
- Lack of concentration
- Poor Memory
- Poor quality performance at school or work
- Lack of motivation or energy
- Headaches or tension
- Upset stomach
- Mistakes/accidents at work or while driving

Prevention

Prevention and treatment of insomnia may require a combination of cognitive behavioral therapy,medications, and lifestyle changes.

Among lifestyle practices, going to sleep and waking up at the same time each day can create a steady pattern which may help to prevent insomnia. Avoidance of vigorous exercise and caffeinated drinks a few hours before going to sleep is recommended, while exercise earlier in the day may be beneficial. Other practices to improve sleep hygiene may include:

- Avoiding or limiting naps
- Treating pain at bedtime
- Avoiding large meals, beverages, alcohol, and nicotine before bedtime
- Finding soothing ways to relax into sleep, including use of white noise
- Making the bedroom suitable for sleep by keeping it dark, cool, and free of devices, such as clocks,cell phones, or televisions
- Maintain regular exercise
- Try relaxing activities before sleeping

Treatments

Cognitive behavioral therapy (CBT): CBT can have beneficial effects that lastwell beyond the end of treatment. It involves combinations of the followingtherapies:

- o **Cognitivetherapy:**Changing attitudes and beliefs that hinder your sleep
- o **Relaxationtraining:**Relaxing yourmind and body
- o **Sleephygienetraining:**Correctingbadhabitsthatcontributetopoorsleep
- o **Sleep restriction:** Severely limiting and then gradually increasing your timein bed

Prescription sleeping pills: Prescription hypnotics can improve sleep when supervised by a physician. The traditional sleeping pills are benzodiazepine receptor agonists, which are typically prescribed for only short-term use. Newer sleeping pills are nonbenzodiazepines, which may pose fewer risks and may be effective for longer-term use.

REFERENCES

[1] The American Academy of Sleep Medicine
[2] **www.aasmnet.org**©AASM2008
[3] Watson NF, Vaughn BV (2006). Clinician's Guide to Sleep Disorders. CRC Press. p. 10. ISBN 978-0-8493-7449-4.
[4] Latterman Family Health Center, 2347 Fifth Ave, McKeesport, PA 15132.

International Journal of All Research Education and Scientific Methods (IJARESM), ISSN: 2455-6211
Volume 10, Issue 9, September-2022, Impact Factor: 7.429, Available online at: www.ijaresm.com

Alice in Wonderland Syndrome

Dr. V. Hemavathy[1], Prof. Girija Baskaran[2], J. Regina Margret Vimala[3]

[1]Principal, Sree Balaji College of Nursing, Chennai
[2]HOD, Dept. Of Medical Surgical Nursing, Sree Balaji College of Nursing, Chennai
[3]M. Sc (N), II Year, Sree Balaji College Of Nursing, Chennai

****

ABSTRACT

Alice in Wonderland syndrome is a disorienting perceptual disorder characterized by discrete episodes of bizarre visual illusions and spatial distortions which has been associated with numerous neurologic and psychiatric conditions. Little is known regarding the electrophysiologic correlates of the visual symptoms described in this syndrome. The authors report the unique case of an 8-year-old boy presenting with visual distortions consistent with Alice in Wonderland syndrome, and an electroencephalogram demonstrating bilateral temporo-occipital slowing which correlated with symptoms of micropsia, teleopsia, and dysmorphopsia.Identification of this clinical syndrome and its electroclinical features are important for establishing a proper diagnosis and subsequent reassurance or appropriate treatment directed toward the underlying etiology.

Keywords: Alice in Wonderland syndrome, teleopsia dysmorphopsia. Microsomatognosia, EEG, paediatric migraine, epilepsy

Alice in wonderland syndrome (AIWS) describes a set of symptoms with alteration of body image. An alteration of visual perception is found in that way that the sizes of body parts or sizes of external objects are perceived incorrectly. The most common perceptions are at night.

The term Alice in Wonderland syndrome (AIWS) was initially coined by John Todd in 1955 to describe some weird somesthetic aura involving the shape or size of the objects and body parts. The name of this disorder was inspired bythe novel of Lewis Carroll and his novel hero Alice. Alice appeared to experience many body size changes throughout the course of the story. Alice even feels her body shrink (microsomatognosia) or growing unexplainably taller (macrosomatognosia) than she actually is. Such visual perceptual distortions may occur in epileptic seizures, encephalitis, drug intoxication, and may be described in patients with schizophrenia or brain lesions. However, migraine and epilepsy are highly involved diseases that cause this type of aural symptoms. In this paper, a unique presentation of a young AIWS patient who has been depressed by experiencing an intermittent perceptual disturbanceof seeing her cat as a huge tiger was reported.

HISTORY

The syndrome is sometimes called Todd's syndrome, in reference to an influential description of the condition in 1955 by Dr. John Todd (1914–1987), a British consultant psychiatrist at High Royds Hospital at Menston in West Yorkshire. Dr. Todd discovered that several of his patients experienced severe headaches causing them to see and perceive objects as greatly out of proportion. In addition, they had altered sense of time and touch, as well as distorted perceptions of their own body. Despite having migraine headaches, none of these patients had brain tumors, damaged eyesight, or mental illness that could have accounted for these and similar symptoms. They were also all able to think lucidly and could distinguish hallucinations from reality, however, their perceptions were distorted.

Dr. Todd speculated that author Lewis Carroll had used his own migraine experiences as a source of inspiration for his famous 1865 novel Alice's Adventures in Wonderland. Carroll's diary reveals that, in 1856, he consulted William Bowman, an eminent ophthalmologist, about the visual manifestations of the migraines he regularly experienced. In Carroll's diaries, he often wrote of a "bilious headache" that came coupled with severe nausea and vomiting. In 1885, he wrote that he had "experienced, for the second time, that odd optical affection of seeing moving fortifications, followed by a headache". Carroll wrote two books about Alice, the heroine after which the syndrome is named. In the story, Alice experiences several strange feelings that overlap with the characteristics of the syndrome, such as slowing time perception. In chapter two of Alice's Adventures in Wonderland (1865), Alice's body shrinks after drinking from a bottle labeled "DRINK ME", after which she consumed a cake that made her so large that she almost touched the ceiling. These features of the story describe the macropsia and micropsia that are so characteristic to this disease.

These symptoms have been reported before in scientific literature, including World War I and II soldiers with occipital lesions, so Todd understood that he was not the first person to discover this phenomenon. Additionally, as early as 1933, other researchers such as Coleman and Lippman had compared these symptoms to the story of Alice in Wonderland. Caro Lippman was the first to hypothesize that the bodily changes that Alice encounters mimicked those of Lewis Carroll's migraine symptoms. Others suggest that Carroll may have familiarized himself with these distorted perceptions through his knowledge of hallucinogenic mushrooms. It has been suggested that Carroll would have been aware of mycologist Mordecai Cubitt Cooke's description of the intoxicating effects of the fungus Amanita muscaria (commonly known as the fly agaric or fly amanita), in his books The Seven Sisters of Sleep and A Plain and Easy Account of British Fungi.

Gulliver's Travels

Alice in Wonderland syndrome's symptom of micropsia has also been related to Jonathan Swift's novel Gulliver's Travels. It has been referred to as "Lilliput sight" and "Lilliputian hallucination", a term coined by British physician Raoul Leroy in 1909.

Alice in Wonderland

Alice in Wonderland syndrome was named after Lewis Carroll's famous 19th-century novel Alice's Adventures in Wonderland. In the story, Alice, the titular character, experiences numerous situations similar to those of micropsia and macropsia. The thorough descriptions of metamorphosis clearly described in the novel were the first of their kind to depict the bodily distortions associated with the condition. There is some speculation that Carroll may have written the story using his own direct experience with episodes of micropsia resulting from the numerous migraines he was known to experience. It has also been suggested that Carroll may have had temporal lobe epilepsy.

In April 2020, a case of Alice in Wonderland syndrome was covered in an episode of the BBC daytime soap opera Doctors, when patient Hazel Gilmore (Alex Jarrett) experienced it.

ANATOMICAL RELATION

An area of the brain that is important to the development of Alice in Wonderland syndrome is the temporal-parietal-occipital carrefour (TPO-C), where TPO-C region is the meeting point of temporooccipital, parietooccipital, and temporoparietal junctions in the brain. The TPO-C region is also crucial as it is the location where somatosensory and visual information are interpreted by the brain to generate any internal or external manifestations. Thus, modificationsto these regions of the brain may trigger the cause of Alice in Wonderland Syndrome and body schema disorders simultaneously.

Depending on which portion of the brain is damaged, the symptoms of Alice in Wonderland syndrome may differ. For example, it has been reported that injury to the anterior portion of the brain is more likely to be correlated to more complex and a wider range of symptoms, whereas damage to the occipital region has mainly been associated with only simple visual disturbances.

CAUSES

Because Alice in Wonderland syndrome is not commonly diagnosed and documented, it is difficult to estimate what the main causes are, if there are any. The cause of over half of the documented cases of Alice in Wonderland syndrome is unknown. Complete and partial forms of the Alice in Wonderland syndrome exist in a range of other disorders, including epilepsy, intoxicants, infectious states, fevers, and brain lesions. Furthermore, the syndrome is commonly associated with migraines, as well as the use of psychoactive drugs. It can also be the initial symptom of the EpsteinBarr virus (see mononucleosis), and a relationship between the syndrome and mononucleosis has been suggested. Within this suggested relationship, Epstein–Barr virus appears to be the most common cause in children, while for adults it is more commonly associated with migraines.

SIGNS AND SYMPTOMS

With over 60 associated symptoms, Alice in Wonderland syndrome affects the sense of vision, sensation, touch, and hearing, as well as the perception of one's own body image. Migraines, nausea, dizziness, and agitation are also commonly associated symptoms with Alice in Wonderland syndrome. Less frequent symptoms also include loss of limb control and coordination, memory loss, lingering touch and sound sensations, and emotional instability. Alice in Wonderland syndrome is often associated with distortion of sensory perception, which involves visual, somatosensory, and non-visual symptoms. Alice in Wonderland syndrome is characterized by the individual being able to recognize the distortion in the perception of their own body and is episodic in nature. Alice in Wonderland syndrome episodes vary in length from person to person. Episodes typically last from a few minutes to an hour, and each episode may vary in experience.

MANAGEMENT

Whenever treatment is considered useful and necessary, it needs to be aimed at the suspected underlying condition. In clinical practice this mostly involves the prescription of antiepileptics, migraine prophylaxes, antiviral agents, or antibiotics. The literature indicates that antipsychotics are rarely prescribed[7] and that in most cases their effectiveness is considered marginal. Moreover, when distortions are experienced as comorbid symptoms in patients with psychosis, it is important to take into account the possibility that they can sometimes be induced or aggravated by antipsychotics because of their potential to lower the threshold for epileptic activity (as has been described for risperidone).

TAKE-HOME POINTS

- AIWS is characterized by perceptual distortions rather than hallucinations or illusions and therefore needs to be distinguished from schizophrenia spectrum and other psychotic disorders
- When symptoms of AIWS are transient and not associated with any other pathology, reassurance that the symptoms themselves are not harmful may suffice
- Based on the large spectrum of known etiologies and the prospect of improved outcome, I recommend auxiliary investigations to address symptom reoccurrence causing major distress or dysfunction, with or without other pathology
- In clinical cases, treatment needs to be directed at underlying conditions

REFERENCES

[1]. https://www.elsevier.es/en-revista-neurologia-english-edition--495-articulo-alice-in-wonderland-syndrome-as-S2173580818301627
[2]. https://en.wikipedia.org/wiki/Alice_in_Wonderland_syndrome
[3]. https://sapienlabs.org/mentalog/the-alice-in-wonderland-syndrome/

International Journal of All Research Education and Scientific Methods (IJARESM), ISSN: 2455-6211
Volume 10, Issue 9, September-2022, Impact Factor: 7.429, Available online at: www.ijaresm.com

Assertiveness

Dr. V. Hemavathy[1], Miss. S. Lavanya[2]

[1]Principal, Sree Balaji College of Nursing
[2]M.SC (N) 2nd Year Student of Sree Balaji College of Nursing

ABSTRACT

Although the concepts underlying assertiveness training have been gaining increasing popularity, the usefulness of the training model to the helping professions was first noted in 1949. Originally conceived as a limited form of behavior Most of the strategies and techniques, however, rest on three basic assumptions about human nature (Percell, 1977):

- **That feelings and attitudes relate closely to behavior;**
- **That behavior is learned; and**
- **That behavior can be changed.**

Key words: Assertiveness, training, behavior.

INTRODUCTION

Assertiveness is one of the most important skills you can learn today. It can be usedin almost any situation at work as well as in your home and social life. Assertiveness changes the way you communicate, changes the way you deal with conflict, and changes your own relationship with yourself. It is the gateway to confidence, respect, and self-esteem. As you will learn in this book, assertiveness is something you are born with and naturally good at. Only the intervention of others with your best interests at heart rob you of assertiveness and teach you unsatisfactory substitutes, such as submission and aggression. But assertiveness isalways waiting for you to re-discover its magic. If you are someone who feels they have lost their way in their relations with others, this session will show you howto claim back your birthright.

What Is Assertiveness?

It is a process, a skill, and a way of behaving. In communicating, it is more easily defined by its absence and its alternative ways of behaving, such as aggression and submission. But Assertiveness is a key quality in all positive and productive relationships and a skill that we should all learn to know better.

One of the skills that takes you to success is self-esteem, the appreciation of your own worth and importance. And Assertiveness is one of the daily habits that will produce self-esteem.
Assertiveness, self-esteem and confidence are inextricably linked.

An Assertive Sequence

There are various ways to resolve a situation where you feel your rights are being infringed without getting angry or giving in. Here is one using the mnemonic LASSIE. It starts with you outlining the situation to the other person, and follows with:

L for Listen to their point of view
A for Acknowledge what they say
S for Say what you honestly think and feel
S for Say what you would like to happen I
for Indicate what the differences are
E for Explore win-win solutions.

Benefits of assertiveness

The reason why Assertiveness matters is that it is the key that unlocks success in so many areas of our lives. In the workplace, it underlies so many of the skills we use in relating to others, such as communication, negotiating, and leadership. In personal relationships, it is the best way to solve problems and man oeuvre our way out of conflict. In ourselves, it is the way to feel good about our lives.

One of the key benefits of Assertiveness is that it helps you eliminate the fear and stress which still today are present in many of our life and work relationships, be they demanding bosses, angry customers, or unhelpful colleagues. Fear and stress-based relationships create different forms of flight-fight reactions in us. These can take the form of avoiding people, giving in to them, battling them, bullying them, or manipulating them. All these routes lead to unease, disease, and ultimate exhaustion. With Assertiveness skills, you learn that fear doesn't have to exist in any relationship you choose to have, whatever the other person wants. Assertiveness gives you back personal control that allows you to act rather than react and to see everyone else the way you see yourself. With love and respect.

Assertiveness is a prime social skill. It may not be as quick at resolving issues as forceful dominance or quiet submission. But it is the route to the most healthy and satisfactory of human behaviors.

Applications of Assertiveness

Many of us don't handle interpersonal relationships well, particularly at work. Instead of feeling good about ourselves, our reactions and responses to others often make us feel tongue-tied and inadequate, on the one hand, and angry and critical on the other. Here aresome of the ways to deal with everyday situations and come out feeling good.

Responding to Compliments

People who have low self-esteem tend to dismiss compliments. Deep down they feel unworthy and are likely to respondto praise with phrases such as, "Who me?" or "It was nothing". You can use three techniques to stop yourself usingsuch self- denigrating replies. First, when someone says something nice about you, simply say "Thanks" in a way that is clear, grateful, and accepting. Secondly, ask people what they liked about what you did.
Thirdly, find something in what they said that you can agree with.

Expressing Your Feelings

A further reason for low self-esteem is the tendency to believe that your views are not as important as other people's. This often happens when you feel you are not as articulate as others in expressing your thoughts and feelings. As a result, you sit and say nothing. This is another trick of your ego to make you feel bad and confirm some old image that you were given as a kid. Put a stop to this and learn to express yourself regardless of what other peoplethink or feel.

REFERENCES

[1] Upgradeurmind.in
[2] Alberti, R.E., & Emmons, M.L. (1986). Your perfect right: A guide to assertive living (5th rev. ed.). San Luis Obispo, CA: Impact.
[3] Clark, C. (1978). Assertive skills for nurses. Wakefield, MA: Contemporary Publishing.

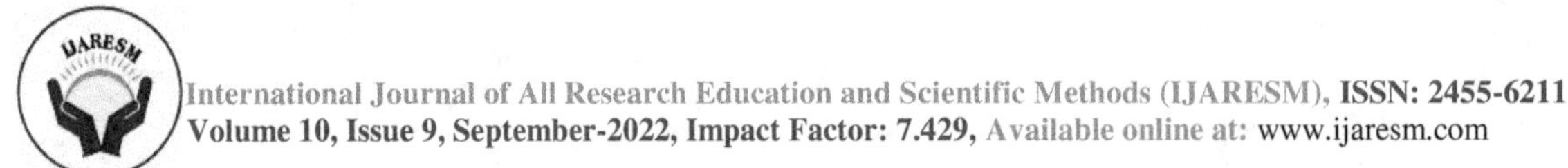
International Journal of All Research Education and Scientific Methods (IJARESM), ISSN: 2455-6211
Volume 10, Issue 9, September-2022, Impact Factor: 7.429, Available online at: www.ijaresm.com

Herlyn-Werner-Wunderlich Syndrome

Dr. V. Hemavathy[1], Dr. Sathyalathasarathy[2], R. Sangeetha[3]

[1]Principal, Sree Balaji College of Nursing, Chrompet, Chennai
[2]HOD, Obstetrics and Gynecology Nursing Dept., Sree Balaji College of Nursing, Chrompet, Chennai
[3]MSc. Nursing, Sree Balaji College of Nursing, Chrompet, Chennai

****

ABSTRACT

HWW syndrome is a very rare congenital anomaly of urogenital tract involving Mullerian ducts and mesonephric ducts. It is characterised by a triad of symptoms - uterus didelphys, obstructed hemivagina and ipsilateral renal agenesis. It presents soon after menarche or shows delayed presentation depending on the type. It can exhibit acute pelvic pain shortly after menarche and may show non-specific and variable symptoms with resultant delay in diagnosis. The most common presentation is pain and dysmenorrhea, and pain and abdominal mass in the lower abdomen secondary to haematocolpos and/or haematometra.

Awareness is necessary in order to diagnose and treat this disorder properly before complications occur. MRI is the preferred modality for the delineation of uterine malformation. When renal anomalies are encountered, a screening should also be made for congenital abnormalities of the reproductive tract and vice versa.

Key words - Uterus didelphys, Vaginal septum, Renal agenesis, Herlyn-Werner-Wunderlich syndrome

INTRODUCTION

The incidence of Mullerian duct anomalies in the literature is estimated to be from 0.5 to 5.0% in the general population. Crosby and Hill in 1962 firstly described the theory of the development of Mullerian ducts. During the embryonic period, The Mullerian ducts (paramesonephric) develop from the coelomic epithelium and grow caudally along the Wolffian ducts (mesonephric) toward the urogenital sinus forming the two uterovaginal canals. At the 11 weeks of gestation, the Mullerian ducts fused laterally to form a single canal which becomes the uterus and the upper tow third of the vagina. Meanwhile, the sino-vaginal bulbs invaginate from the urogenital sinus and meet the caudal end of the fused Mullerian ducts to form the vaginal plate. Finally, the vaginal plate is reabsorbed and being canalized to form the lower part of the vagina. This process of resorption is completed by the 24 weeks of gestation. Defective of fusion, or failure of resorption of the inferior portions of the Müllerian ducts during early embryological life results in uterus didelphys (double uterus) or septated uterus. The vagina may beseptated as well. Uterus Didelphys occurred in about 0.16% of fertile women. The coincidence of Renal agenesis on the same side of the obstructed vagina can be explained by an embryologic arrest at 8 weeks of pregnancy, simultaneously affecting the two neighbors: The Mullerian (paramesonephric) and Wolffian (metanephric) ducts.

Purslow CE in 1922, firstly described a case of a young woman with regular menstruation had gradually increasing pelvic pain and appearance of a pelvic mass after menarche. MOSTYN P. and EMBREY B. in 1950 described a case of obstructed Hemi-vagina and a uterus didelphys as well as an ipsilateral renal anomaly. While Herlyn and Werner in 1971 initially described the syndrome as blind hemi-vagina with ipsilateral renal agenesis, finally, Wunderlich in 1976 added the bicornuate uterus as a feature of the syndrome.

Nowadays, Herlyn-Werner-Wunderlich syndrome (HWW), represents a complex female genital malformation with uterus didelphys, unilateral low vaginal obstruction, and ipsilateral renal agenesis.

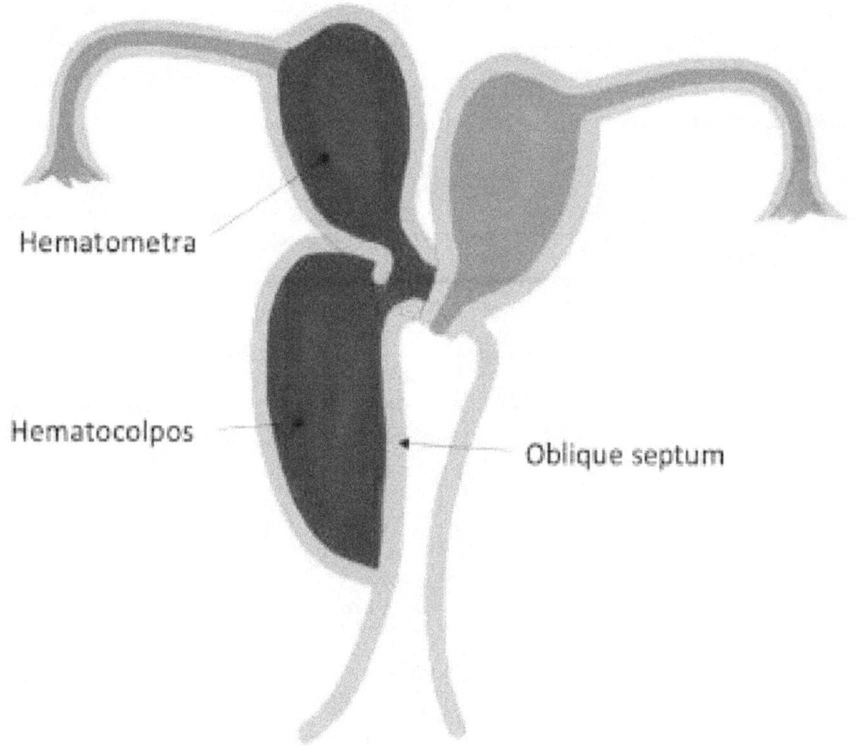

SIGNS AND SYMPTOMS

Patient with (HWWS) usually becomes symptomatic after menarche. Having two normal uterus and obstructed hemivagina, the patient will have regular menses through the non-obstructed vaginal side which coincides with a cyclic pelvic pain (dysmenorrhea) from the encumbered blood in the obstructed vaginal side, that leads to hematometra, hematocolpous and retrograde menstrual flow, which explains the increased prevalence of endometriosis, pelvic adhesions and retention of urine in these patients. A ten years review of this anomaly showed that (73%) of patients presented with dysmenorrhea, (71%) with pelvic or paravaginal mass.

Lan Zhu, et al. proposed New Classification of Herlyn-Werner-Wunderlich Syndrome based on a complete or incomplete obstructed hemivagina

DIAGNOSIS

Diagnosis of HWWS is usually confirmed by sonography and magnetic resonance imaging (MRI). Sonography can detect the pelvic cystic mass and may detect the uterine malformations.However, MRI provides more detailed information regarding the uterine contour, the shape of the intrauterine cavity and its continuity with each vaginal lumen, the character of the septum, and the nature of the fluid content, as well as the presence of the associated aspects such as endometriosis, or renal anomalies.

Many associated Urological malformations have been described with HWWS including, renal duplication, multicystic dysplastic kidney and renal agenesis which is the most commonly reported associated urologic anomaly.

Herlyn-Werner-Wunderlich Syndrome

Class	Class 1 Completely obstructed hemivagina		Class 2 Incompletely obstructed hemivagina	
Subclass	1.1 Blind hemivagina	1.2 Cervicovaginal atresia without communicating uteri	2.1 Partial reabsorption of the vaginal septum	2.2 With communicating uteri
Findings	Completely obstructed hemivagina; uterus behind the septum is completely isolated from the contralateral uterus with no communication between the duplicated uterus and vagina	Completely obstructed hemivagina; cervix behind the septum is maldeveloped or atretic	Small communication exists between the 2 vaginas; uterus behind the septum is completely isolated from the contralateral uterus	Later age of onset, presents years after menarche; purulent or bloody vaginal discharge; can present with ascending genital infections
Clinical feature	Hematocolpos; hematometra, hematosalpinx; hemoperitoneum; endometriosis; secondary pelvic adhesions; pyosalpinx; pyocolpos	Clinical features similar to the patients as in Class 1.1	Small communication exists between the duplicated cervices	Menstrual blood drainage is still impeded

TREATMENT

Treatment is surgical, with resection of the septum dividing the two hemivaginas in order to relieve the obstruction. Subsequent successful pregnancy in the obstructed uterus has been reported.

COMPLICATIONS

The potential complications of this syndrome are pyohematocolpos or pyosalpinx, which may lead to pelvic peritonitis. While long-term complications are endometriosis, pelvic adhesions leading to chronic pelvic pain, and infertility. Which require early diagnosis and treatment of this syndrome in order to avoid theses complications and to preserve the fertility. Therefore patient affected by (HWWS) needs further follow up to predict these possible complications.

The clinical manifestations and age of onset may differ among the different types of Herlyn–Werner–Wunderlich syndrome (HWWS). Ultrasound is recommended for early screening and MRI, for further diagnosis. Early diagnosis and surgical treatment may help to avoid further complications; however, it should be noted that inflammation and swelling may render the surgery difficult and reduce its success rate.

REFERENCES

[1] https://radiopaedia.org/articles/herlyn-werner-wunderlich-syndrome?lang=us
[2] https://clinmedjournals.org/articles/ogcr/obstetrics-and-gynaecology-cases-reviews-ogcr-6-156.php
[3] https://jmedicalcasereports.biomedcentral.com/articles/10.1186/s13256-019-2258-6/figures/8
[4] https://www.ncbi.nlm.nih.gov/pmc/articles/PMC3139160/
[5] https://www.sciencedirect.com/science/article/pii/S1930043321003514
[6] https://www.sciencedirect.com/science/article/pii/S193004332100457X

International Journal of All Research Education and Scientific Methods (IJARESM), ISSN: 2455-6211
Volume 10, Issue 9, September-2022, Impact Factor: 7.429, Available online at: www.ijaresm.com

Prader Willi Syndrome

Dr. V. Hemavathy[1], Mrs. V. J. Binipaul[2], Miss. R. Bhavani[3]

[1]Principal, Sree Balaji College of Nursing
[2] H.O.D., Professor, Sree Balaji College of Nursing
[3] M.Sc (N) IInd Year Student, Sree Balaji College Of Nursing

****

ABSTRACT

Prader-Willi syndrome (PWS) is a highly variable genetic disorder affecting multiple body systems whose most consistent major manifestations include hypotonia with poor suck and poor weight gain in infancy; mild mental retardation, hypogonadism, growth hormone insufficiency causing short stature for the family, early childhood-onset hyperphagia and obesity, characteristic appearance, and behavioral and sometimes psychiatric disturbance. Many more minor characteristics can be helpful in diagnosis and important in management. PWSis an example of a genetic condition involving genomic imprinting. It can occur by three main mechanisms, which lead to absence of expression of paternally inherited genes in the chromosome 15 region: paternal microdeletion, maternal uniparental disomy, and imprinting defect.

Key words: Prader Willi Syndrome, Disomy, Hypogonadism, Hypotonia

DEFINITION

Prader-Willi syndrome (PWS) is a disorder caused by a deletion or disruption of genes in the proximal arm of chromosome 15 or by maternal disomy in the proximal arm of chromosome 15. Commonly associated characteristicsof this disorder include diminished fetal activity, obesity, hypotonia, intellectual disability, short stature, hypogonadotropic hypogonadism, strabismus, and small hands and feet.

INCIDENCE

Prader–Willi syndrome (PWS) is a rare genetic disorder with a birth incidence of 1/10,000 to 1/30,000.

CAUSE

Prader-Willi syndrome is a genetic disorder, a condition caused by an error in one or more genes. Although the exact mechanisms responsible for Prader-Willi syndrome havenot been identified, the problem lies in the genes located in a particular region of chromosome 15.Prader-Willi syndrome occurs because certain paternal genes that should be expressed are not for one of these reasons:

- Paternal genes on chromosome 15 are missing.
- The child inherited two copies of chromosome 15 from the mother and no chromosome 15 from the father.
- There's some error or defect in paternal genes on chromosome 15.

PATHOPHYSIOLOGY

At birth, growth parameters, such as weight, length, and body mass index, are 15 to 20% smaller in patients with Prader Willi Syndrome than those of their unaffected siblings, indicating that the growth is irregular during the prenatal period. Hypotonia prenatally causes decreased fetal movement, an abnormal position at the time of the delivery leadingto increased cesarean and assisted birth.

SIGNS AND SYMPTOMS

Signs and symptoms of Prader-Willi syndrome can vary among individuals. Symptoms may slowly change over time from childhood to adulthood.

In Infants

Signs and symptoms that may be present from birth include:

- Poor muscle tone
- Distinct facial features
- Poor sucking reflex
- Generally poor responsiveness
- Underdeveloped genitalis

In Early childhood to adulthood

Other features of Prader-Willi syndrome appear during early childhood and remain throughout life, requiring careful management. These features may include:

- Food craving and weight gain
- Underdeveloped sex organs
- Poor growth and physical development
- Cognitive impairment
- Delayed motor development
- Speech problems
- Behavioral problems
- Sleep disorders
- Other signs and symptoms: These may include small hands and feet, curvature of the spine (scoliosis), hip problems, reduced saliva flow, nearsightedness and other vision problems, problems regulating body temperature, a high pain tolerance, or a lack of pigment (hypopigmentation) causing hair, eyes and skin to be pale.

DIAGNOSIS

Typically, doctors suspect Prader-Willi syndrome based on signs and symptoms. A definitive diagnosis can almost always be made through a blood test. This genetic testing can identify abnormalities in child's chromosomes that indicate Prader-Willi syndrome.

TREATMENT

Early diagnosis and treatment can improve the quality of life for people with Prader-Willi syndrome.

Good nutrition for infants: High-calorie formula or special feeding methods to help the baby gain weight and will monitor the child's growth.

Human growth hormone (HGH) treatment: It is called somatropin is used to treat children with Prader-Willi syndrome. Somatropin is given by daily injection.

Sex hormone treatment: Hormone replacement therapy (testosterone for males or estrogen and progesterone for females) to replenish low levels of sex hormones.

Other treatments: These may include addressing specific symptoms or complications identified by eye exams for vision problems, tests for hypothyroidism or diabetes, and examinations for scoliosis.

REFERENCES

[1]. Akefeldt A, Tornhage CJ, Gillberg C. A woman with Prader-Willi syndrome gives birth to a healthy baby girl. DevMed Child Neurol. 1999;41:789–90.

[2]. Bischof JM, Stewart CL, Wevrick R. Inactivation of the mouse Magel2 gene results in growth abnormalities similar to Prader-Willi syndrome. Hum Mol Genet. 2007;16:2713–9.

[3]. Butler MG, Lee J, Manzardo AM, Gold JA, Miller JL, Kimonis V, Driscoll DJ. Growth charts for non-growth hormone treated Prader-Wili syndrome. Pediatrics. 2015;135:e126–35.

[4]. Cassidy SB, Driscoll DJ. Prader-Willi Syndrome. Eur J Hum Genet. 2009;17:3–13.

[5]. Horsthemke B, Buiting K. Imprinting defects on human chromosome 15. Cytogenet Genome Res. 2006;113:292–9

International Journal of All Research Education and Scientific Methods (IJARESM), ISSN: 2455-6211
Volume 10, Issue 9, September-2022, Impact Factor: 7.429, Available online at: www.ijaresm.com

"An Experimental Study to Assess The Effectiveness of Assertiveness Training on Self Esteem Among Early Adolescents Studying in Hilton Matriculation Higher Secondary School, Chrompet"

Dr. V. Hemavathy[1], Miss. M. Ranjini[2]

[1]Principal Sree Balaji College of Nursing
[2]M.Sc (N) 2nd Year Student Of Sree Balaji College of Nursing

****

ABSTRACT

Assertiveness is the ability to express yourself and your rights without violating the rights of others. Assertiveness is frequently misunderstood. Non -Assertiveness involves expressing thoughts, feelings and beliefs in a way that is inappropriate and violates the rights of others while assertiveness tries to find a solution.Assertiveness is tool for confidently and way of saying „Yes" or „No" . Personal identity is mainly basedon the self – concept. Self –concept is the cognitive or thinking component of the self, and generally refers to the totality of a complex, organized, and dynamic system of learned beliefs, attitudes and opinions that each person holds to be true about his or her personal existence.The last and best component of self-concept is self – Esteem.Lack of self-esteem may lead to poor acquisition of the skills and abilities that are needed to achieve objectives and thus it turns affect one"s successful way of life.Assertiveness training is a form of behavior therapy designed to help people stand for themselves-to empower themselves, in more contemporary terms and helps in improving self-esteem.

Key words: Assertiveness, self-esteem, assertiveness training

OBJECTIVES

- To assess the level of Self-Esteem among early adolescents studying in Hilton matriculation higher secondary school.
- To evaluate the effectiveness of Assertive training on Self-Esteem among early adolescents studying in Hilton matriculation higher secondary school.
- To associate the level of Self-Esteem among early adolescents studying in Hilton matriculation highersecondary school, with their selected socio demographic variables.

METHODOLOGY

A pre-experimental one group pre-test–post-test design was used in this study. The research was conducted at Hilton matriculation higher secondary school-chrompet with the sample of 60 early adolescents.A non-probability sampling (Purposive sampling) technique was used in this study.The tool used for the study was Rosenberg Self-Esteem Scale.

RESULT

In the pretest majority of the early adolescents 42 (70.0%) had low level of Self-Esteem, 18 (30%) had average level of Self-Esteem and no one had high self-esteem in the pretest. In the post test (After Intervention-Assertiveness Training) majority of the adolescents 38 (63.3%) had high level of Self-Esteem, 22 (36.7%) had average level of Self Esteem.Thepre -test mean Self-Esteem score was 13.18 with theStandard Deviation 1.86, whereas post-test mean Self-Esteem score was 24.57 with aStandard Deviation 1.92. Mean Difference is 11.38.The student paired 't' test was done to find out the difference between the pre-test and post test score, 't' value 30.84 was greater than the table value which wassignificant at 0.001 level. This shows that the difference in the score was due to theintervention (Assertiveness Training) and also this proves that the AssertivenessTraining was effectivein increasing the Self-Esteem among adolescents studying inselected school.

CONCLUSION

Assertive training helps in boosting self-confidence ,creates winning situation and gain a sense of empowerment ,moreover it is cost effective ,non pharmacological therapy that promotes self-esteem among early adolescence .

REFERENCES

[1]. Ahuja Niraj (2002) A Short text book of psychiatry 1st edition ,New Delhi, Jaypee publishers.[2]. BT Basavanthappa (2000) Nursing research 2nd edition ,Bangalore, Jaypee publishers.
[3]. https://eujournal.org.
[4]. https://scholar.google.co.in.

www.ingramcontent.com/pod-product-compliance
Lightning Source LLC
LaVergne TN
LVHW060830170826
845678LV00010B/1942

* 9 7 8 9 3 9 5 7 7 3 1 7 1 *